Desktop Yoga™

Desktop Yoga™

*The Anytime, Anywhere Relaxation Program
for Office Slaves, Internet Addicts, and
Stressed-Out Students*

JULIE T. LUSK, M.ED., LPC
Certified Yoga Teacher

A PERIGEE BOOK

As with all exercise programs, please consult your physician before beginning. These exercises are not intended to replace medical care. The creators, producers, publishers, distributors, and author disclaim any liability or loss in connection with the exercises or advice herein.

A Perigee Book
Published by The Berkley Publishing Group
A division of Penguin Putnam Inc.
375 Hudson Street
New York, New York 10014

First edition: November 1998

Published simultaneously in Canada.

The Penguin Putnam Inc. World Wide Web site address is
http://www.penguinputnam.com

Library of Congress Cataloging-in-Publication Data

Lusk, Julie T.
     Desktop yoga : for office slaves, internet addicts, and stressed-out students / Julie T. Lusk.
        p.   cm.
     "A Perigee book."
     Includes bibliographical references.
     ISBN 0-399-52446-0
     1. Yoga, Hatha.   2. Stress management.   3. Relaxation.   4. White collar workers—Health and hygiene.   I. Title.
RA781.7.L86   1998
613.7'046—dc21   98-19187
                                                                      CIP

Printed in the United States of America

10 9 8 7 6 5

Dedicated to mouse potatoes and those glued to the keyboard, chained to the chair, and otherwise stiffened by the workstation.

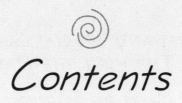

Contents

Acknowledgments

*D*esktop Yoga has been an extraordinary adventure and one I'll never forget. I often felt as if this project was blanketed with blessings and good fortune all along the way. It is my hope that Desktop Yoga will inspire others to discover the beauty of yoga and explore all its exciting possibilities for personal and professional growth and well-being.

There are many people who deserve my heartfelt thanks for all their time, energy, expertise, feedback, and support. Special thanks are extended to my husband, David, who believes in me and always gives me love and encouragement. Angie Tapin, my mom, gave me the vision to succeed and do my best. My brother Tom taught me to dream big, and my sister Mary Noel showed me how to overcome obstacles with grace and grit. My dad, rest his soul, would have been so proud.

My yoga teachers have a special place in my heart for sharing their knowledge and wisdom with me. I am especially grateful to Tracey Rich, Ganga White, Lilias Folan, Joe Panoor, Swami Satchidananda, Nischala Devi, and all my friends at Yogaville. My yoga students have challenged me to keep learning and growing and sharing the spirit of yoga.

Acknowledgments

Many, many friends have helped me directly and indirectly and I wish I could name all of them. Belleruth Naparstek, Judy Bates, Deb Kern, Becky Laney, Aileen and Erica Pandapas, Greg Law, Sallie Garst, Nola Mabry, Dave Robertson, Jim Strohecker, Diana Amato, Richard Miller, Bill Hettler, Roger Jahnke, Kim Carroll, Jane Hoover, Kathleen and Bill Baudreau, Shirley Rosien, Michael Arloski, Karen Early, Judy Fulop, Lou Castern, Jeni Brasher, Jenifer O'Leary, Paul Linden, Mangala Warner, Charles MacInerney, Bill Andersen, the Seekers, and Swami Sarvaananda have all given me ideas, information, and inspiration.

This book would not have been possible without the professional help of Loretta Barrett, Dolores McMullan, Marian Montgomery, Hal Bates, and James Hiney. I am especially grateful to Kathleen Kelly-Hoffman for being loyal to this project and for her wonderful drawings.

Introduction

*J*ust like your computer screen needs a screen-saver to keep it from burn-ing out, your body needs a body-saver. Sitting in one position and staring at your work for hours on end will cause you to have an achy back and cramped wrists and hands. Before you know it, your body is stiff and creaks when trying to move, your eyes are dry and bloodshot, and your legs have gone to sleep. When this happens, your mind, thoughts, and creativity soon become dull, lifeless, and boring. No fun, in other words, and life is meant to be fun.

The information age and its tools are here to stay. Nearly every occupa-tion and numerous hobbies rely on computers, faxes, scanners, and E-mail. The internet has become many people's primary source of information, com-munication, and entertainment. These developments are transforming the way we work and how we spend our free time. It is possible to send letters, conduct research, run a business, plan a trip, exchange information, do your banking, play a game, and shop without leaving your computer desk.

Along with all the rewards and benefits of the computer age, there are risks and problems as well. Computer work causes physical wear and tear on your muscles, tissues, and nerves. Sitting still for long periods of time and repeating the same limited keyboard and mouse movements over and over again can lead to stiffness, pain, fatigue, numbness, tingling, irritation, swelling, and soreness. In the worst case scenario, long-term damage can be done to your wrists, back, shoulders, neck, and eyes. In fact, the United States Bureau of Labor Statistics reports that over 60 percent of all workplace-related injuries can be attributed to repetitive stress injuries. This is costing businesses billions of dollars in medical costs and lost productivity.

Not only can extended and improper computer use create physical problems, it can be mentally draining and intimidating as well. This is especially true if you don't feel comfortable using a computer or are using a new system or software program.

Have you ever gotten trapped by what you're doing so that precious time slips by? Simply hacking away, just focused on what you're doing, not even blinking. Somehow you've become stuck in some sort of desktop daze and now you can hardly move because you haven't lifted anything but your fingertips for hours.

On the bright side, you have been focused and entered a timeless place and become one with what you're doing, which is developing the wonderful skill of concentration. Perhaps, you might be interested in taking this ability to concentrate a step further, and learn to meditate. Meditation will calm you down, replace your scattered feelings with centeredness, and make you a better problem solver by bringing your intuition and inner wisdom out of hiding. Feelings of peace, balance, meaning, and purpose are a few rewards from meditation.

Emotional stress and imbalance can also result from computer work. At one point or another, I'll bet that you have felt a wide range of emotions associated with computer work. Have you ever felt frustrated, irritated, confused, or on the verge of smashing something? On the other hand, feelings of accomplishment, achievement, satisfaction, fun, and even joy can also be experienced.

Hatha yoga is an ancient system of breathing techniques and physical postures that are done standing, sitting, or lying down. It is known to enhance health, reduce stress, and create physical flexibility, tone, strength, and stamina. Yoga increases physical, mental, and emotional awareness and cultivates feelings of mindfulness, wholesomeness, and relaxation.

Desktop Yoga has been developed to give you relief from the aches and pains of computer and sedentary working conditions. Traditional yoga postures and breathing techniques have been modified so they can be done while sitting in a chair at the office without any other special equipment or clothing. It's a new and different way to apply the principles of yoga and its priceless lessons to modern-day life. It's user-friendly!

Learning Desktop Yoga will reward you with simple things you can do to remain relaxed, comfortable, and productive. This book is intended to help you develop strategies, attitudes, and specific stretches to help you cope with the computer world. It will prompt you to take action so you aren't victimized and tortured by your work any longer. More important, you will have energy and vitality at the end of your workday to dedicate to your personal life.

part one

Desktop Yoga

one

Desktop Yoga Basics

"*Y*oga" is the Sanskrit word for union. This union refers to the spiritual practice of cultivating awareness and balance within the mind, body, emotions, and the creative self. Too often people feel fragmented because the mind is going in many different directions at the same time. The body is being ignored or crying out for attention, the emotions are exploding or perhaps being stifled, and the creative self is forgotten. Learning to listen to and respond to each of these aspects brings about a connected feeling. Experiencing this sense of connection will enable you to live more fully and more completely.

Desktop Yoga is designed to bring relief to your aching body and relaxation to your scattered self when you need it most—at work. It can be done right in your chair without any special equipment and is especially useful for people wearing ties and/or hose and pumps. T-shirts and jeans work well too. Desktop Yoga can be done anytime or anyplace.

—at the keyboard (computer, piano, organ, use your imagination)

—by the copier or fax machine

—when stuck in traffic and at stoplights

—in trains, planes, and cars

—while on hold

—during television commercials

In other words, at work, home, and at play.

Desktop Yoga is different than most types of exercise and stretching programs because it is a form of movement done mindfully. Activities such as stretching, aerobics, swimming, running, or using exercise equipment can usually be done without having to concentrate on what you are doing. In fact, most people purposefully let their minds wander and will often listen to music in order to distract themselves from the physical activity.

Moving mindfully means that you focus your attention on the sensations of the movements. In other words, you remain aware of the feelings associated with each posture on a moment-to-moment basis. Where do you feel muscular tension and which stretches would provide relief? Which muscles are being stretched? Are you stretching too much or too little? Are you moving too quickly?

One of the things that makes Desktop Yoga so delightfully different than simply stretching is the special emphasis that's placed on full and complete breathing. The increase of fresh oxygen to the bloodstream will bring a fresh ability to think clearly and focus. It will develop a special awareness and honest responsiveness to your body's needs and foster a felt sense of emotional well-being. Each moment blossoms and comes vibrantly alive.

Your body has the ability to heal itself from many of its problems. Anything you can do to support and enhance this natural ability is most important. Yoga supports the healthy functioning of the body, mind, and spirit. Yoga restores flexibility and mobility as it improves circulation, nerve and gland efficiency, stamina, energy, and breathing capacity.

The present moment comes alive when you synchronize and balance your breath with your physical movements. Doing this offers mental clarity and can help you feel calm and collected.

You need not be flexible or young to do yoga. Yoga is built upon a foundation that honors and respects your own natural skills and abilities. Regular practice brings inner and outer flexibility, strength, and coordination.

All the systems of the body benefit from the practice of yoga, and yoga ensures the healthy, balanced functioning of these systems. The benefits that follow will be enhanced if you imagine these things happening as you breathe. This gives you a way to turn your natural tendency to daydream into something that can actually make a significant difference to your well-being.

Systems for Moving and Standing

Skeletal System

Your skeletal system consists of 206 bones to provide the framework for your body and to protect your internal organs. The bones act as a storage area for minerals. Blood vessels and nerves supply your bones with nutrients and oxygen and the marrow of certain bones produce red blood cells and some white blood cells. Ligaments, the connective tissues, are also a part of the skeletal system.

The maintenance of a sturdy bone structure is essential to being able to enjoy a long and healthy life. Regular exercise, proper nutrition, and certain hormones are needed to keep the skeleton strong. Yoga contains many weight-bearing postures to facilitate this process.

Joints help make movement possible and exist wherever two bones meet. Yoga increases blood supply to your joints and yoga movements give them the opportunity to move and stretch. This will definitely help you maintain and improve your mobility. Yoga will help you keep from getting stiff from age and lack of movement.

Muscular System

All of us have three types of muscles. Skeletal muscles are attached to the bones to enable the joints to twist and bend. The cardiac muscle forms the powerful wall of the heart, and smooth muscles control the movements of the digestive, circulatory, urinary, and reproductive systems.

Exercise is needed to keep your muscles healthy. The problem is that many sports and other exercises tend to shorten and contract certain muscles or concentrate movement on a small number of muscles, which increases stiffness.

Yoga, on the other hand, fosters flexibility and suppleness because it encourages you to take the time to stretch most of your muscles and ligaments in a slow and smooth manner. Doing so relieves stored tensions and stretches and lengthens muscles, achieving good tone. Having flexibility will decrease the possibility of injury from sports and exercise and will more than likely improve your performance as well. Longer muscles are much more efficient than shorter ones.

Muscles can retain memories of mental, emotional, and physical stress that can create ongoing problems. Fortunately, these memories can be released through the practice of yoga poses. Bodywork, such as massage, can also help.

Systems for Energy and Disposal of Waste

Digestive System

The teeth, tongue, esophagus, stomach, intestines, liver, and pancreas make up the digestive system.

The digestive system transforms your food into the fuel that is needed for nourishment, energy, and for the growth and repair of cells. Eating proper types and amounts of food is an important part of yoga.

Various yoga poses stimulate digestion by systematically compressing and releasing the intestinal tract. Organs such as the alimentary canal, stomach, intestines, and liver all benefit from yoga. Compressing the right side of the abdomen before the left side while doing yoga is thought to assist in the digestive process. Because of the shape of the colon, food moves through your system more effectively for maximum assimilation and decreases the risk of internal congestion. This helps remove wastes from the system through proper elimination.

Respiratory System

The respiratory system both supplies oxygen to your entire body and removes carbon dioxide and other gaseous wastes. Ineffective breathing that is shallow, or irregular harms all other bodily functions by decreasing the functioning of the cells, organs, and glands. Poor oxygenization decreases concentration and memory while increasing mental fatigue.

Yoga emphasizes deep diaphragmatic breathing which improves the functioning of the lungs, stimulates the cardiovascular system, and aids digestion and elimination. Breath is considered to be the life force in yoga and is directly related to mental, physical, and emotional balance.

Cardiovascular and Circulatory Systems

Your heart pumps blood through the vessels to all parts of the body. It carries nutrients, antibodies, oxygen, and hormones to the cells. Your circulatory system also helps regulate body temperature.

Yoga postures help nourish all parts of the body by improving and increasing the flow of oxygenated blood throughout the body. Internal tissues, organs, and glands are much healthier with proper blood supply. Yoga increases blood flow and strengthens the heart. Yoga even increases the elasticity of the arteries. These benefits are achieved by doing the yoga movements gradually and without force. Inverted postures are particularly helpful to the circulatory system since the effects of gravity on the body are reversed. The following chapter, Breathing Basics, goes into further detail about respiration and breathing.

Systems for Coordination and Control

Nervous System

Your central nervous system is made up of your brain, the spinal cord, and the nerves. The brain constantly monitors internal and external stimuli and sends and receives messages from your muscles, glands, and other organs. Your spinal cord carries messages between your brain and the lower parts of your body. It also acts as a reflex center. Thoughts, emotions, and memories also stem from the nervous system.

The goal of many yoga postures is to improve alignment, flexibility, and strength to the back. Another goal is to increase the circulation to the spinal column and the nerves associated with it. Yoga is well-known for its ability to prevent backaches and relieve back pain. Inverted postures increase the circulation to the brain. A healthy respiratory system has a highly beneficial effect on the brain and nervous system.

Endocrine System

The endocrine system is composed of glands that regulate the hormones. The major glands are the hypothalamus, pineal, pituitary, thyroid, parathyroid, thymus, genital, pancreas, and adrenals. These glands regulate hunger, thirst, sleep, wakefulness, body temperature, sex drive, menstruation, growth, metabolism, insulin production, lymph activity, the flight or fight response, emotions, and keeps the mineral and water levels in balance.

Yoga poses help to strengthen the endocrine system through exercise. Yoga postures influence most glands by irrigating them with increased blood flow through alternately compressing and releasing them.

Integumentary System

The skin is the largest organ of the body. It keeps renewing itself throughout life and grows faster than any other organ. It protects you from harmful bacteria, extremes in temperature, sunlight, and other outside threats. It's waterproof and elastic. Some skin is tough and other skin is thin. Your skin is a storehouse for fats and glycogen and also manufactures vitamin D when it's exposed to sunlight.

Yoga increases the blood flow to the skin, which helps its complexion, tone, and color. The skin is stretched by yoga, which improves its elasticity. Last but not least, yoga delays the formation of wrinkles and the effects of aging on the skin.

Sensory System

Your eyes, ears, nose, tongue, and other sense organs report to your brain what is going on in and around you. These organs bring us pleasure as well as warn us about danger. Yoga improves the circulation to all of the sense organs, which helps them function properly. Your tongue serves the digestive system and your nose serves your respiratory system. Yoga eye movements stimulate and exercise the eye muscles, which enables them to stay healthy and strong.

System for Producing New Life

Reproductive System

The primary purpose of the male and female reproductive systems is to create new life. Sexual well-being and satisfaction is dependent on freedom of tension, a relaxed attitude, good muscle tone, proper functioning of the glands and circulation, flexible limbs and joints, and an efficient nervous system. Yoga practice enhances all of these functions.

System for Greater Awareness

The Pranic System

Prana is considered to be the life force and one of the foundations of yoga practices. This life force is called *chi* in China and *ki* in Japan. It is continuous and sustains life. The breath is thought to be the primary source of prana; however, it is also found in food and other earthly elements. Prana exists inside and outside the body and is the basis for energy, clarity, health, and vitality.

A lack of prana results in restlessness, inertia, apathy, and a feeling of being stuck. This happens when prana is being unnecessarily dispersed outside the body and is not being kept within. Prana can be regulated by the quality of your breath as well as your mental condition. In fact, breathing patterns influence the mind and the mind influences the breath.

Yoga directly improves the quality of your prana through the many breathing techniques that can be learned and practiced. In turn, your mental state will benefit greatly. You may notice an increase in your ability to concentrate, focus, remember, and think clearly.

two

Breathing Basics

Your breathing plays a very special and important role in yoga and in the overall health of your body, mind, and emotions. All this tends to soothe the spirit as well. Breathing "yogically" sets yoga apart from other forms of exercise.

Breathing fully and completely gives you mental clarity and physical endurance. Your cells, organs, glands, and tissues will benefit greatly.

When breathing in, your lungs fill with blood waiting to be oxygenated. Once oxygenated, the blood then circulates throughout your body cleansing, refreshing, and purifying your cells, all the while picking up poisons, toxins, and waste that are released when you breathe out. As the diaphragm expands on the in-breath, it massages the abdominal organs, aiding digestion and elimination.

Shallow unrhythmic breathing disrupts this process. This leads to sluggish functioning of the cells and a destructive dullness throughout your entire physical, mental, and emotional system.

Diaphragmatic breathing is done by breathing in deeply enough that the belly area feels as if it is expanding. In fact, your belly will literally rise and fall as breaths are taken. Doing so slows the heart rate and is associated with normal blood pressure. It increases lymphatic flow and the transfer of oxygen from the blood to the tissues. Diaphragmatic breathing improves venous return of the blood to the heart and normalizes blood flow in the lungs. It also dilates the brain and coronary arteries, which increases blood and oxygen to the brain and heart. It lowers tension and stress in the muscles and can reduce the sensation of pain. Diaphragmatic breathing enhances vitality, energy, self-awareness, and stability.

A natural stress release is created as you breathe diaphragmatically. Your heartbeat will naturally slow down as your diaphragm stimulates the vagus nerve. Your overall circulation will also improve.

Tips

Breathe in and out through your nose. Your nose is designed to prepare the air for your lungs by warming or cooling it, moisturizing it, and removing dust particles and other small debris that is contained in the air.

Your lungs are large and meant to be used. Give yourself a chance to breathe all the way in and all the way out. It's important to take your time to breathe fully and completely.

Since a decent breath begins with a complete exhalation, start by breathing out through your nose as much air as you can. Even after you think all the air has been released, squeeze a bit more out. You will notice a big difference in your lung capacity if you will first push as much air out as you possibly can. This will automatically prepare your lungs for a full and complete breath.

Breathe in through your nose smoothly and evenly so that the air fills up the lowest part of your lungs first. Then let it expand to the midsection and finally to the uppermost part of your lungs.

Breathe all the way back out again. Let the air release from the top to the bottom.

To get the hang of it, gently place your hands on your tummy so that the tips of your middle fingers slightly touch each other. As you breathe in, notice how your fingertips will slightly separate. Your fingertips will go back together when you breathe back out. This happens when your diaphragm expands and gently massages the abdominal area.

Be mindful of your shoulders. If you feel any tightness or tension, let them relax and soften as you exhale.

Try focusing your attention on the sensation of breathing itself. Know when you are breathing in. Know when you are breathing out. When your mind drifts away, gently bring your attention back to your breath.

Notice the gentle caress of a steady and even in-breath and the sense of freedom and release generated with a slow out-breath. Let the exhalation be an outlet for any unwanted physical, emotional, or mental sensations.

Rhythmic breathing is important. It influences the mind, calms the emotions, and relaxes the nerves. Have you ever noticed what happens to your breathing as your emotional states change? Next time you feel irritated, notice how shallow and irregular your breath becomes. On the other hand, feeling relaxed and at ease calms, lengthens, and smooths out the rate of breathing.

First, practice breathing so that your inhalations and exhalations are smooth, even, and of the same length. In other words, begin counting to yourself as the air fills your lungs up and then breathe out for that same number of counts. Let one breath flow into the next without any jerks. After this becomes easy, you can begin to let your exhalation last a little longer than your inhalation.

Maintain a complete, full, smooth breath during yoga. As you learn how to do the postures, gradually begin to coordinate your breathing with your movements. You will breathe in when you open up and stretch and you will breathe out when you bend. Let your breath and body create a synchronized rhythm to bring a conscious awareness to the mind/body/breath balance. You can get a natural high whenever you want.

Here are some special breathing techniques to practice.

1. Ujjayi (pronounced "ooo" as in cool, "ji" as in hi) breathing helps you concentrate and calm down, and builds heat, endurance, and stamina. It will help you establish control over the breath and will extend the amount of time that it takes to inhale and exhale. A longer breath slows down the heartbeat. Ujjayi is especially good for reducing stress, improving digestion, and toning the nerves.

Although you will always breathe in and out through your nose when doing Ujjayi, it will be easier to learn if you first breathe in and out through your mouth while whispering "haaa." Doing so will allow you to experience an open feeling in your throat. Next, close your mouth and continue breathing while maintaining that feeling in your throat. When done correctly, there is a slight constriction in the glottis (the opening between the vocal chords) during inhalation and exhalation. Ujjayi breath creates a unique, audible Darth Vader–type sound.

2. Three-Part Breathing or Three-Fold Breathing will reward you with all the benefits of diaphragmatic breathing. Not only will it relax you, it will also replenish your energy and enable you to use your lungs fully and completely.

Begin by releasing all the air from your lungs through your nose. Use your abdominal muscles to help squeeze all the air out.

Slowly and smoothly breathe in through your nose so you can feel your belly filling followed by an expansion around your entire rib cage (front, back, and sides). Finally, allow the air to fill the collarbone area.

Let all the air be released slowly through your nose as you empty your lungs as completely as possible from the top to the bottom.

Continue three-part breathing for as long as you comfortably can.

As always, try to keep your attention placed on your breathing. Each time your mind wanders, simply bring your attention back to your breath. The more you practice, the easier it will become to improve your lung capacity, hold your focus, and increase the number of breaths you can take without becoming distracted.

3. Releasing Breath. Get your anger and frustrations out with the help of your breath. It will also clean, strengthen, and stimulate the lungs.

Breathe in through your nose and forcefully breathe out through your mouth. This is even more effective if you compress your abdominal muscles on the out-breath. Imagine your anxious feelings being sent out each time you breathe out.

4. Alternate Nostril Breathing tends to calm, balance, and regulate energy levels both physically and subtly. Did you know that scientists have discovered that each side of the brain is dedicated to different functions? In most people, the right hemisphere (side) of the brain fosters your abstract,

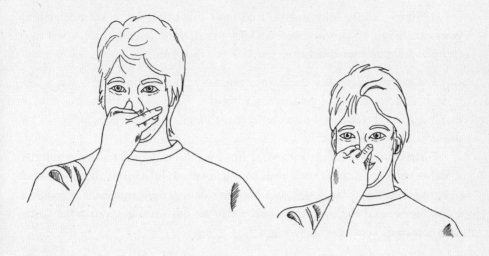

creative, and emotional nature, while logical, rational, and numeric thinking is accomplished on the left. Energetically breathing through the right nostril facilitates and intensifies the activity of the body and mind, and breathing through the left nostril has a cooling and receptive influence. If you pay attention, you will notice a shift in dominance between your nostrils as you breathe. In other words, air flows more smoothly on one side at a time. This shift usually occurs every sixty to ninety minutes. Alternate nostril breathing helps balance this natural cycle while purifying the subtle nerve channels, and stimulating the brain wholistically. It is also a fantastic remedy for headaches, and is very effective at reducing the effects of stress. Mental clarity is enhanced.

Here's how. Take your right hand and bend your pointer and middle fingers towards the palm. Gently place your thumb against your right nostril and breath out from your left nostril. Ujjayi breathing is recommended.

Breathe in through the left side as much as possible and then close the left nostril with your ring and pinky fingers while you release your thumb from the right nostril to release the air. Breathe in that same side (right) and then gently press your thumb against the right nostril, release the ring and pinky fingers, and send the air out the left side. This completes one round. Continue switching sides for several more rounds and end by breathing out from the right side. Sixteen rounds is ideal.

At first, practice breathing so that your inhalation is the same length as your exhalation. When this becomes easy to do, try to let your exhalation take twice as long as your inhalation.

5. Cooling Breath is great for when you are hot under the collar. Likewise, it will literally cool you off on a hot day. Along with all the benefits of diaphragmatic breathing, this technique is thought to be particularly good for the eyes, ears, and throat.

Form a small opening with your lips by rolling the sides of your tongue together to create a tube. Stick your tongue out and inhale through the round opening. Breathe in as if you are drinking cool refreshing water through a straw. Slowly and evenly, breathe the warm air out through your nose. Continue on until you have cooled down.

6. Mindful Breathing is easier said than done. Mindful breathing will increase your concentration and reduce nervous tension.

Simply observe your breath as you breathe naturally. Don't try to change the rate, rhythm, sound, or depth of your breathing. Just notice the physical sensations of breathing. You will soon perceive the coolness of the in-breath and the warmth of the out-breath. Take time to notice how your lungs and ribs expand and contract with each breath. Each time you become distracted, and you definitely will, simply return your attention back to the breath.

7. Aromatic Breathing is delightful and as refreshing as a pleasant vacation. Imagine you are breathing in your favorite fragrances. For example, imagine breathing in the smell of freshly baked bread, an ocean breeze, the scent of a cozy campfire, flowers, cinnamon, clouds, fried onions, popcorn, or the fragrance of springtime. Let your imagination run free.

three

Getting Started

*D*esktop Yoga is going to work wonders for you. Not only will you be able to avoid many of the aches and pains of working at a computer, sitting at a desk, or leaning over a workbench or microscope, you will feel much better at the end of the day and have enough energy to enjoy your personal life and interests. You will also begin noticing a shift in attitude that will reduce stress and bring a sense of enjoyment to living in the present moment, no matter where you are or what you are doing.

To get the maximum return on your investment, however, it is equally important to pay attention to your actual desktop and to develop the proper approach to practicing yoga. You will defeat the benefits of doing Desktop Yoga if your workstation is poorly designed and your posture is bad. In other words, no amount of neck stretches will work if you have to crane your neck all day to view the monitor.

Adjust your workstation as follows:

—Ideally, your computer screen should be an arm's length away from your eyes. If necessary, have your bifocals adjusted so you can look at your screen comfortably without neck or eye strain.

—Adjust the computer screen; it should be just below eye level so that you can look down upon it. This will help save your neck.

—Situate your screen to avoid glare. Use window curtains, blinds, or shades if needed.

—The screen is a dirt magnet and dust is tiring to your eyes. So wipe it off on a regular basis.

—The computer keyboard should be located at elbow level.

—Choose a chair that is padded, firm, and has a waterfall edge.

—Adjust your chair so it both fits your size and supports your back and legs properly. Your chair should be wider than your thighs.

—Adjust your chair or the height of your desk so your forearms are horizontal to the floor.

—Face your work directly and keep your things within easy reach.

—Place your document holder at the same level and distance as the screen to cut down on having to shift your head and neck back and forth constantly and to cut down on eyestrain.

Adjust your posture as follows:
—Your upper arm and forearm should form a right angle (ninety degrees).

—Your forearms should be parallel to the floor.

—Keep your arms close to your sides.

—If possible and comfortable, support your elbows on the arms of your chair.

—Keep your wrists straight; use a wrist rest for support. Avoid resting your wrists or arms on sharp edges.

—Your back should be kept in an "S" shape and not a "C" shape.

—Your legs should not touch the underside of your workstation. You may need to take the drawer out.

—Your thighs should be parallel to the floor.

—Keep both feet flat on the floor and use a footrest if your legs are short or your chair is too big.

—Use a headset if you spend a lot of time on the phone.

—Take regular breaks. Walk around as often as possible.

Adjust your work space as follows:
—If possible, reduce the amount of unnecessary noise in your area since excess noise is jarring to the nervous system. Could you close the door, move a loud printer or copier, or adjust the volume on the intercom or music? You may also want to take your breaks in a quiet place.

—Decorate your area with some beautiful plants. Not only will they add some life, they will help remove carbon dioxide from the atmosphere and improve air quality. In fact, we breathe in oxygen and release carbon dioxide while plants take in carbon dioxide and release oxygen.

B. C. Wolverton, Ph.D., a scientist with the National Aeronautics and Space Administration (NASA), has conducted research and discovered that some plants are better than others at purifying the air. Golden pothos, areca palm, and dracaena "Janet Craig" are all recommended as overall air cleaners. Formaldehyde, the most pervasive indoor toxin, can be taken care of with Boston ferns, Kimberley queen, florists' mum, or English ivy.

Cultivating the Proper Approach to Practicing Desktop Yoga

Yoga's rewards will be diminished without the proper approach to practicing the movements. Without the proper attitude, Desktop Yoga will be reduced to ordinary stretches that will be limited in usefulness. As you probably already know, attitude is everything, and Desktop Yoga will give you practical tools to improve yourself.

Here are some tips to help you get the most out of Desktop Yoga. As you get better at integrating these principles into your yoga, you will notice a nice shift occurring in your approach to nearly everything you do. You'll feel more comfortable in your body, your thinking and concentration will improve, your emotions will settle down, and life will feel balanced.

—Do what you can do; never force. This means that if you can comfortably bend over twelve inches, you shouldn't bend fifteen or eight inches.

—Always remember to breathe deeply and fully (refer to chapter 2).

—Balance your movements. If you stretch to the right, follow it with a stretch to the left. When you bend forward, remember to bend backward next.

—To help with digestion and elimination, remember to compress, bend, or otherwise move your right side first, and then the left. It will feel better if you wait a while to practice yoga after eating a heavy meal.

—Hold each pose for as long as is comfortable—not too long and not too short. Pay attention and respond to the signals that your body sends.

—Try to do yoga on a regular basis in order to receive maximum benefits. It is much more valuable to take a brief three-to-five-minute Desktop Yoga break every thirty minutes than it is to try to find time to spend thirty minutes on it all at once. Taking yoga breaks throughout the day will help you remain relaxed and in control.

—Be aware of the signals that your body sends to you throughout the day. Learn to relax your eyes, neck, shoulders, and back before you get that headache.

—If you have high blood pressure, do *not* hold your arms overhead with straight or stiff elbows. Always keep a soft bend in the knees instead of stiffening and straightening them, as these positions raise the blood pressure.

—It's better to do a move once or twice so you can keep your attention focused on what you are doing, rather than to repeat or hold something so long that you lose your concentration.

—Yoga is meant to be "interesting." It is not meant to stroke your ego with compliments nor is it meant to criticize it with curses. When this happens, as it often will, simply bring your attention back into the moment and accept whatever is happening.

four

Neck and Shoulders

Your neck is often abused and taken for granted. Not only does it have to hold your head up all day long, it gets stiff, cranky, and out of line when you make it hold the phone between your ear and your shoulder. Sitting at a computer or hunching over a desk throws your neck and head off balance, which can lead to head and shoulder aches.

Shoulders and necks are well-known for holding up the weight of the world. We "shoulder responsibility" and "stick our necks out." They often hold a lot of tension and become stiff as a board. Constant computer hacking brings the shoulders forward, which cramps the lungs and heart. The following movements can help prevent the repetitive motion injuries described in chapter 13.

Here are some simple things you can do for your shoulders and neck. They can be done either sitting or standing. Most of them can even be done at a stoplight.

1. Neck Stretch. These stretches will prevent stiffness in the neck and shoulders, improve circulation, and cultivate flexibility in the neck area.

Sit up tall and allow your shoulders to relax. Try not to round your shoulders forward. Let your right ear float toward your right shoulder. Only move it as far as you comfortably can without force. Take a few full breaths. Just when your muscles get tired, take a breath in and bring your head back up to the center.

Next, let your left ear move toward your left shoulder and take a few breaths. Then, bring your head back to center on an in-breath. It is common for one side to feel more limber than the other side.

Moving your head from side to side can be repeated several times. While doing this, imagine all the stress and strain that's held around your neck releasing and letting go.

Next, let your chin glide down to your chest and take a few breaths. Remember to let it go as far as it comfortably can without stress or strain. When ready, bring your head up to center.

Do not move your head backward. It puts too much stress on the vertebra located in the back of the neck.

2. Neck Movements will limber the neck and cervical spine, increase circulation, and prevent headaches that are felt at the back of the head and neck.

Let your right ear float slowly to your right shoulder. Keep your shoulders down and relaxed. Then, slowly and smoothly roll your head forward and to the left. Just make a semicircle. Next, move your head from the left back to the right.

Repeat these semicircles several times and remember to breathe. See if you can notice that your neck tension is dissolving and feeling better. Don't make a full circle, as this creates too much neck strain.

For a different stretch, move your chin so that it is over your right shoulder. Move your chin down toward your shoulder. Please don't strain.

Slowly and smoothly, roll your chin in a semicircle toward your chest until it is resting in the center, and then look down. Take time for a few long breaths in this position—your neck will receive the benefits of the extra stretch, and your thyroid will be gently massaged.

Continue moving your chin to the left shoulder. Rest and breathe.

Circle your chin back around to the front. Rest and breathe. And then over to the right shoulder.

For maximum benefit, these movements can be repeated three to five more times.

3. Infinity Neck Stretches will increase the flexibility in the neck, improve circulation, relieve stress, and stretch your eye muscles.

Lower your shoulders and let them relax. There's no need for unnecessary tension. Begin drawing the infinity symbol (a sideways figure eight) with your nose. Trace the pattern with your eyes as you stretch. Practice this several times in a row.

Next, see if you can do it just as smoothly in the opposite direction. Imagine your creativity stretching in infinite directions.

4. Neck Flex. With these movements, your shoulders, neck, and spine will become limber, circulation to your neck and upper back will improve, and muscular tension will begin to dissolve.

Clasp your hands behind your head and stretch your elbows out to both sides. Slowly twist your head, neck, and elbows gently to the right. Look at your right elbow and take a few breaths.

Slide your head, neck, and arms back to the center and then toward the left. Only move as far as you comfortably can. Gaze at your left elbow as you breathe evenly and smoothly. When your mind begins to wander, bring your attention back to the stretch and to your breath. It's okay to repeat these moves several times, but don't forget to breathe.

If you are less flexible, keep your chin parallel to the floor and lower your arms and hands to your sides. Simply turn your head to the right as slowly and steadily and as far as possible. You can extend the stretch by looking to the right with your eyes. Breathe.

Next, move your chin back to center and then over to the left side. Don't forget to stretch your eyes to the left.

Come back to center and rest.

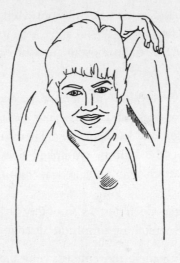

5. Elbow Up. These movements will stretch the arms and shoulders, increase circulation, and tone the arm muscles.

Point your right elbow toward the sky with your arm and hand moving down toward the middle of your back. Place your left hand on your extended elbow and gently pull it to the left. Hold for a few breaths as you notice the wonderful stretch to your right shoulder.

Bring both arms down to your sides and wiggle your arms and shoulders around in all directions.

Now, send your left elbow straight up with your left arm and hand going down your back. Put your right hand on your left elbow, take a breath, and pull softly to the right. Apply just enough pressure so that you feel a nice stretch to your left shoulder.

Lower your arms and wiggle them around some more.

6. Shoulder Sway. Use these stretches to increase flexibility and circulation in the arms, shoulders, and neck. It causes a gentle twist in the upper back muscles and relieves muscular tension.

Hold both arms straight out in front of you and level with your shoulders. Take a few breaths as you gaze at your fingertips.

Bend both arms at your elbows and place each hand on the opposite elbow. Your arms are still shoulder high. Breathe out as you sway your arms to the right side (keep your torso motionless). Breathe in as you sway your arms back to center. Breathe out, swaying your arms to the left. Breathe in as you move them back to center and breathe out again as they smoothly move to the right. Keep moving and breathing like this for several more rounds.

7. **Shoulder Shrugs** are done to reduce shoulder tension, relieve stress, and increase the suppleness in the shoulders and upper back.

Let your arms and shoulders relax at your sides. Bring both shoulders up toward your ears while you breathe in through your nose. Breathe out through your mouth as you let your shoulders drop back down. Really let go. It's fine to repeat this a few more times. Frustrations as well as shoulder tension will be released.

8. **Shoulder Rolls** will loosen the shoulder joints, stretch the upper back muscles, and improve your posture.

This time, form a complete circle with your shoulders by bringing them up toward your ears. Move them backward, feeling a squeeze between your shoulder blades, and then move them all the way down and then toward the front and up again. Repeat these circular movements while letting your arms and hands relax. Remember to breathe.

In yoga, we always move in both directions. So this time, start with your shoulders as low as they go. Next move them backward, up, and around front. This is done smoothly, evenly, and gently, just like your breathing.

9. **Shoulder Wings** will improve your circulation in the upper body and stretch your shoulders and arms. Respiration will deepen.

Rest your right hand on your right shoulder and your left hand on your left shoulder. Begin slowly and evenly flapping your arms as if they are wings. Increase the tempo and let your imagination take flight and soar.

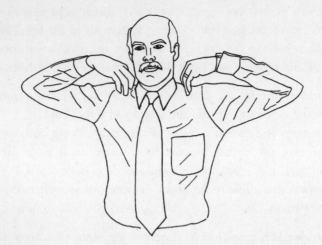

10. Taking Flight. These movements will tone the muscles in your arms, stretch the shoulders, and improve circulation and concentration.

Let your arms fall to your sides and take a few deep breaths. Turn your hands away from your body and breathe in as you raise your arms overhead until your fingertips touch. Turn your hands around so your palms are touching and breathe out as you lower your arms back to your sides. Continue moving your arms up and down a few more times.

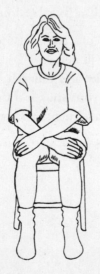

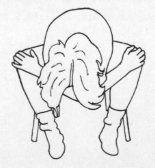

11. Shoulder Stretch. This stretch will relieve muscular tension from the base of your spine up through your shoulders. It relieves back strain and feels great.

Begin by uncrossing your legs. Place both feet flat on the floor about twelve inches apart. Bend forward with care and put your right hand on your left knee and your left hand on your right knee. (Ladies, be sure to face a wall or private area if you are wearing a skirt.)

Slowly move your knees away from each other and as far apart as is comfortable. Feel the wonderful stretch to your shoulders and back.

12. Energy Stretch. The range of motion in your upper body will improve, your energy will increase, and concentration and respiration will be enhanced.

Place both feet on the floor and let your arms hang to your sides. As you breathe in slowly, begin raising your arms straight out in front of you until they are shoulder height. Let your shoulders relax and be sure not to lift them up. Still breathing in, bring your arms out to both sides and then raise them over your head until your palms touch.

Breathe out as you lower your arms back down to your sides. Continue on for several deep, diaphragmatic breaths.

The trick here is to raise your arms during the time it takes to breathe in and to lower your arms during the time it takes to breathe out. Experiment with the speed to keep your arm movements synchronized with the rate and rhythm of your breath. Practice makes perfect.

five

Face

Your face probably gets more of a workout from tension than you may realize. It's no wonder that there are so many expressions for the stress that is felt in and around the face: work and fellow employees can make you want to "pull your hair out" and "raise an eyebrow or two," which causes you to have to keep a "sharp eye on things." Do you know people who "keep a stiff upper lip," have to "chin up," or "grin and bear it?" Instead of breathing fully, do you "nose around," "sniff things out," and "keep your nose to the grind?" Have you ever had to "bite the bullet?"

With all due seriousness, computer screens torture your eyes, which can cause them to become tired and dry in no time at all. Poor lighting, glare, dry air, and constantly staring at the monitor all contribute to eyestrain. Chances are good that it's hard to recognize how exhausted your eyes are until your head aches. Here are a few preliminary steps you can take to avoid such strains:

—If possible, adjust the screen colors so they aren't too hard on your eyes; try soft colors for a nice change.

—Avoid glare by choosing a place for your computer that doesn't reflect windows or lights.

—Remember to look away from your screen every fifteen minutes or so. It's too hard on your eyes to do such close work without a break.

1. Eye Movements. After a while, eye muscles tire out and it becomes harder to focus. To prevent this from happening, you can practice these eye movements. They will strengthen your eye muscles and eyesight and stimulate the brain. Do them sitting up, standing, or lying down.

Start doing the eye movements slowly and pick up the pace after you can do it smoothly without jerks. Pay more attention to the eye movements than to the visual effects. Try not to feel any skips to any parts of the circle as your eyes are moving round and around. Remember to keep your head still as you do all the eye movements. Let your facial muscles relax as well.

First Variation: Up and Down. With your head and neck evenly aligned and movement-free, look up as far as you can and try to see up and over your head. Then look down as if you would like to see under your chin. Keep doing this several times in a row. Follow this by bringing your eyes back to center and blink them a couple of times. Afterward, rest with your eyes closed and take several deep breaths.

Second Variation: Side to Side. This time look quickly to the right and try to see behind your ear, then rapidly look to the left and try to see behind your left ear. Keep looking back and forth several times. When finished, bring your eyes back to center. Blink a few times and rest them with your eyes closed.

Third Variation: Clockwise. Begin by looking at "twelve o'clock," then to one o'clock, two o'clock and on around until you get back to twelve o'clock. Keep circling for five to ten complete rotations. Rest when you are through.

Fourth Variation: You guessed it, move your eyes in a counterclockwise direction for several rounds.

Fifth Variation: Trace a sideways figure eight (∞) from side to side several times. Finish by bringing your eyes back to center and then close your eyes to rest them.

2. Palming will rest and relax your eyes, calm your nerves, and quiet your mind. Your respiration will increase as long as you remember to breathe deeply and fully.

Rub your hands rapidly together with your palms and fingers touching. Keep rubbing until you feel the generation of some heat and energy. Next, rest your elbows on your desk. Cup your hands and gently place them over your closed eyes. Let the warmth and darkness soothe your eyes. Take several long and easy breaths as you imagine the tiredness being released with your out-breath and energy and vitality returning with your in-breath.

Note: If somebody catches you doing this, be prepared to say something clever like, "Can't a person even pray around here?" Your other option is to tell them what you're doing and have them join in.

3. Nose Wiggles will tone your facial muscles and nourish your complexion with better blood flow.

Pretend that a bug has landed on your nose. Wiggle it off by moving your nose all around.

4. Bridge Work reduces muscular tightness, increases circulation, and relieves headaches.

Softly pinch the bridge of your nose and massage the area between your eyebrows. This will help you relax.

Rub your forehead with your fingers and smooth the tension away. It feels fantastic to make circles at the temples. Remember to breathe.

Be creative.

5. Ear Rub. Take both your hands and begin to rub, press, pull, fold, and massage your ears. This will stimulate the nerve endings that are found on the outside surface of your ears.

Surround your ears with your fingers by making a "V" with your pointer and middle fingers. Rub your fingers up and down, pressing firmly. Be sure to unclench your teeth.

Notice the warmth that is generated by doing the ear rub.

6. Ear Taps increase hearing acuity.

Cup your left hand over your right ear and tap it several times with the fingertips of your right hand. Then, cup your right hand over your left ear and tap it using the fingertips of your left hand.

Avoid ear taps if you are wearing a hearing aid.

7. Soothing Sounds. Take a break from noise pollution to calm the mind and soothe the nervous system. Turn the computer, printer, and radio off, forward your calls, and shut the door. Focus your attention by taking a few calming breaths. Bring your attention back to your breath when your mind wanders.

Imagine listening to some of your favorite sounds. Can you hear the sound of popcorn popping, a babbling brook, a roaring waterfall, melodious wind chimes, a crackling fire, the steady rhythm of a beating heart, or a cat purr? Imagine the sound of a piano, drums, flute, or trumpet. Enjoy the sounds of silence—floating clouds, the shining sun, a beautiful seashell.

8. Big Mouth. Lots of people hold tension in the area of the jaw. If it gets bad enough, a chronic problem may develop called TMJ (Temporomandibular Joint Syndrome). Practicing big mouth will relieve muscular tension and your facial muscles will tone up.

Open and close your mouth over and over. Then quickly move your jaw sideways to the right and left. Finally, mix the up and down movements with the side-to-side movements. Sideways movements are not recommended for anyone who already has TMJ because the jaw could become locked.

9. Mouth Swishers will tone your facial muscles, relieve tension, and improve circulation.

Fill your cheeks up with air and swish it all around. Poke it into all the nooks and crannies inside your mouth. Pretend you are rinsing with a refreshing mouthwash.

10. Tongue Time improves circulation and is fun.

Massage the inside of your mouth with your tongue. Spend time massaging your cheeks, the roof of your mouth, inside your lips, and around your teeth and gums. Go ahead, stretch your tongue out as far as it will go. Let your tongue soften inside your mouth when through.

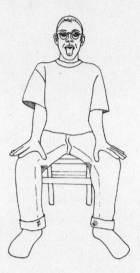

11. Lion Pose. This lovely pose will release frustrations as it brings a fresh supply of blood to your eyes, sinuses, and complexion. It's also good for your throat and voice box, which helps sore throats and voice strain.

Sit with both your feet flat on the floor and place your hands on your knees. Now, take a big deep breath in as you bug out your eyes, stick your tongue way out, and stretch out your fingers. You can either hold your breath the whole time or you can release it along with a natural sound as you make the lion face. You'll notice a refreshing tingling feeling in your face, which is thought to work like a natural face-lift.

12. Smile.

six

Arms, Wrists, and Hands

Arms and hands are almost perpetual motion machines and don't get the respect and attention they deserve. Fingers go, go, go and get into all sorts of things. Repetitive stress injuries, like carpal tunnel syndrome, have created a crisis in the workplace. Not only is it very painful to the person who suffers from it, it is also very costly to businesses and industry. Yoga has been shown to provide relief for this menacing condition.

Here are some yoga moves to help your arms, wrists, and hands.

1. Reach for the Stars. These stretches will limber and tone your arms, shoulders, and spine.

Bring both arms over your head and keep them raised while reaching upward. First stretch your right arm a little further and reach for the stars. Next, let the right side relax a bit as the left side reaches up. Feel the stretch throughout your upper body, shoulders, sides, arms, and fingers. Of course, you are breathing in unison with your stretches.

2. Heart Opener. These movements will improve circulation, stimulate the thymus gland, and increase your energy.

This time, form your hands into fists and begin to tap your fists all along your heart and chest. Continue tapping your shoulders, and then move the motions around to your back. When you are warmed up, pound a bit harder and faster.

3. Open Your Wings improves respiration and strengthens and stretches your arms and shoulders.

Begin by placing your open hands upon your chest. Can you feel the beating of your heart?

Breathe in fully as you unfold your arms and stretch them out to both sides. Breathe out as you let your hands float back to your chest.

Continue opening and closing your "wings" as you breathe. Air comes in as you open your wings up and the air goes out as your wings close.

4. Strong Arms. This strengthens and tones your arms while it lengthens your back and relieves your bottom.

Place your hands beside yourself on your chair seat and hold on to the sides of your chair. Press down to raise yourself up into the air. Hold yourself up from your chair for a few deep breaths. Lower your bottom onto the chair. Rest, and then repeat several more times.

5. Circle Around. Do these movements to loosen, limber, and improve the range of motion in your shoulders. Your arms will tone up, and your upper back, chest, and mid-back will be opened and stretched.

Hold your arms out from your shoulders and spread your fingers. Begin making small circles in a forward direction. Gradually increase the size of the circles until they are as large as possible.

Change directions and gradually decrease the circle size until they become small again.

Lower your arms and take a couple of full breaths while you rest a few moments. Repeat the circular movements from the opposite direction.

6. Air Swimming. These movements will increase circulation, improve range of motion, and improve the flexibility of your arms, shoulders, and upper back.

Rotate your arms in large circles as if you are swimming forward. Reverse the direction and swim backward.

7. Wrist Rolls will increase circulation while stretching and toning your wrists, hands, and lower arms.

Let your arms rest at your sides and circle your wrists and hands round and round. First circle around one way, and then in the opposite direction. This will improve your circulation and flexibility.

8. Hand Helpers. These stretches will tone and stretch your hands, wrists, and arms. Circulation will improve as well.

First make a tight fist and feel the tension. Then, let all the tension be released. Repeat.

Stretch your fingers and palms out as much as you can. Take your time to feel the stretch. Let your hands and fingers relax gently upon your lap for several moments.

Hold your arms out in front of you with your palms facing the floor, and bend your wrists so your fingers point to the sky. Next, point them toward the earth. Repeat, and don't forget to breathe.

9. Hand Shake. This will relieve muscular tension, increase circulation, and reduce blood pressure.

Shake your arms and hands vigorously. Make believe that you are trying to shake off some sticky stuff that has stuck to your fingers. Feel the energy vibrations spreading throughout your being.

10. Hand Rub. Rub and massage one hand with the other to improve circulation and reduce muscular tension. Remember to rub your wrist, palm, and each finger. Repeat on the other side.

11. Cow Face. These movements will open and stretch your shoulders and chest, improve your posture, and stimulate the nerves at the base of the spine.

Sit up straight and reach your right arm over your head and bend it at the elbow so it goes down the center of your back. Next, bring your left arm down to your side and bend it at the elbow so it reaches up the center of your back. Hold your fingers together. If you can't reach, don't force. Just hold a towel, sock, or necktie instead. As you hold, you can look up toward your right elbow. When done, let your arms return to your sides and sway and shake them gently.

For the other side, reach your left arm over your head and bend it at the elbow so it goes down the center of your back. Next, bring your right arm

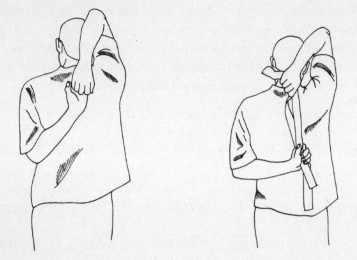

down to your side and bend it at the elbow so it reaches up the center of your back. Hold your hands together. While breathing and holding your fingers, look up to your left elbow. Finally, let your arms go back to your sides and sway and shake them gently. Now, isn't that better?

Don't be surprised if one side is more flexible and easier to stretch than the other. With practice, your flexibility will improve.

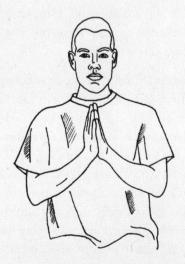

12. Namaste. *Namaste* is a Sanskrit word that means "I honor the light within you." People from India say namaste to one another instead of hello and good-bye. In my book, it sure beats "Hi, how are ya?" and "See ya later."

Touch the palms of your hands and your fingers together at the center of your chest and near the area of your heart. Doing so will help you slow down, calm your mind, soothe your spirit, and help you feel more centered and grounded.

Take your time to feel the skin touching. Notice the temperature of your hands.

Take a few quiet breaths. What else can you sense?

Begin rubbing your hands briskly against each other until you feel some warmth and energy.

Slowly begin to separate your hands, and feel the energy and heat between your hands. Notice how far you're able to separate your hands and still feel this energy.

Rub your hands again to generate more warmth and energy. Smooth this newfound energy wherever it hurts. Let it soak in and comfort you. Honor the light and energy.

Finish by holding your palms together and quiet yourself down with several deep diaphragmatic breaths.

seven

Back

*D*ifficult work is often described as "backbreaking," and although it is meant as a figure of speech, just ask any employer about the cost of workers' compensation claims stemming from back injuries. Taking care of your back by using good mechanics and keeping it strong and flexible can prevent this needless suffering.

As with all the movements contained in this book, always remember how important it is to move at your own ability. Try not to overdo or underdo a stretch. It also helps if you breathe out when you bend forward and breathe in when you open and stretch out.

The following postures will relieve back strain by increasing the circulation and strengthening the muscles in the area surrounding the vertebrae. You'll also notice an improvement in your posture.

1. Sitting Well. Good posture is one of the most important ingredients for a healthy back. Poor posture is not only tiring, it creates unnecessary work for your muscles and ligaments, restricts your capacity to breathe, constricts circulation, and interferes with digestion.

Do yourself a huge favor and take some time to learn the proper way to sit. Don't get discouraged at first if it feels awkward and uncomfortable, it's just that your back muscles have become weak from your former bad habits. In time, your back will become strong, flexible, and healthy again. Sitting properly involves your feet, sit bones, spine, shoulders, neck, and chin.

First of all, sit on your sit bones instead of slouched over with your weight resting on your tailbone. The sit bones are the curved boney ridges at the lower portion of your pelvis. To find them, sit on an unpadded chair and slip your hands between the chair and your buttocks. Do you feel the sit bones? Rock back and forth a bit until you feel the most weight and pressure from the sit bones on your hands. This is the area that you are supposed to sit on. This places your pelvis in an upright and central position and will support your pelvis, spine, neck, and even your head.

Sit away from the back of the chair with your feet flat on the floor. Place your feet and knees hip-width apart. It's best if your knees are a bit lower than your hips.

Sit on your sit bones. Go ahead, try sitting on your hands first in order to get used to where your sit bones are located. Experience the difference it makes to the feeling of your spine.

Align your shoulders by pulling them up near your ears, and circle them around back so you can feel a squeeze between your shoulder blades. Let your shoulders drop down and leave them alone. While you're at it, relax your arms and hands by releasing all tension and tightness.

Lengthen your back to relieve spinal compression by lifting gently up and out of your pelvis. This is done by raising up from your rib cage instead of from your shoulders.

Feel the area from your pelvis, ribs, and chest opening up and lengthening. Make sure that your shoulders are still down and relaxed.

Stretch the back of your neck by lowering your chin and head. Raise your head slowly so that the crown of your head is pointing straight up to the sky. Adjust your chin so that it is horizontal to the floor and isn't jutting out or pulling in. Notice the space between your shoulders and ears.

Unclench your teeth and let your tongue soften.

Let your weight settle and sink back onto your sit bones.

You will sometimes want to use the back of your chair for support. Instead of sitting on your tailbone and slouching into a curved "C" shape, be sure to sit on your sit bones and scoot all the way back until the base of your spine is against the back of the chair.

2. Forward Fold. This delightful stretch will limber up and stretch your arms, rib cage, shoulders, and entire spine. Circulation to your head and brain will increase and the abdominal organs will receive a massage.

Push your chair a little ways out from your workstation and sit toward the front of the chair. (If you don't, you'll bump your head on your desk and it will hurt. Pain has *no* place in yoga.)

Place your feet flat on the floor and about eight to twelve inches apart. Next, clasp your hands behind you and at the small of your back. Straighten your elbows and begin stretching your arms up and away from your body. Only bring them up to a comfortable distance and be careful not to strain your elbows.

Feel the squeeze between your shoulder blades and notice how your shoulders and chest are stretching and expanding. Take a couple of nice, deep, smooth breaths.

Now, as you exhale, begin folding forward from your hips so that your upper body is resting on your lap. Continue to breathe long, full breaths. Let your head hang and raise your arms up even higher. After you've had enough, breathe in as you sit back up, and finally lower your arms back to your sides.

The forward fold is illustrated in the Seated Sun Salute on page 72.

3. Seated Cobra will open up your rib cage and shoulders as it tones, stretches, and strengthens your entire back and shoulder area. Your kidneys, adrenal glands, and abdominal organs will be massaged, which will help your digestion.

Sit on your chair with both feet flat on the floor and take several diaphragmatic breaths. Face the wall if you are wearing a skirt.

Place your hands on your knees and slowly bend forward until your chest is resting on your lap. Exhale as you bend forward.

Spread your knees and feet so that your hands are directly under your shoulders. Position yourself so that your head, neck, and back are in a straight line. Look toward the floor.

Slowly bring your chin forward. Breathe in and begin lifting and curving your head up. Let your torso remain resting on your lap, elongate your spine, and begin raising your shoulders up. Please don't strain.

Breathe out and slowly, and steadily lower your shoulders and upper body back down.

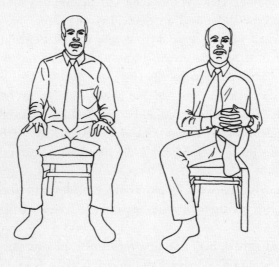

4. Wind Reliever. This easy stretch will relax and limber your lower back, hips, and legs. Digestion and elimination will improve.

Sit on your chair with both feet flat on the floor and take several diaphragmatic breaths. Face the wall if you are wearing a skirt.

Slowly and easily, bring your right leg up with your knee bent. Hold your shin with your hands as you press it up against your torso and hug. As you continue breathing deeply, you will create a wonderful abdominal massage. This is especially good for the organs on the right side, such as your gall bladder, liver, and right ovary (if you have the latter). Lower your foot slowly to the floor.

As usual, you'll always stretch out both sides. This time, slowly and smoothly, bring your left leg up with your knee bent. Hold it with your hands as you press it up against your torso, and hug. Continue breathing deeply. This stretch is especially good for the organs on the left side, such as your pancreas, spleen, and left ovary (if you have one).

Always remember to hug the right side first and then the left. Doing so will help encourage proper digestion and elimination.

5. Seated Side Twist. This important pose will increase the flexibility and circulation to the entire spine and improve your eyesight by massaging and stretching the eye muscles.

Either place both feet flat on the floor with your feet, knees, and thighs together, or put your right leg over the left. Take your left hand and place it on the outside of your right knee and press gently. Keep your left arm extended.

With your back straight, lift your chest and slowly begin turning to the right. Start the twist from the waist and then move your chest, shoulders, neck, and finally your eyes. Take your other arm (right) and put it around your back near your waist. Breathe in as you lengthen your back and breathe out as you twist. Release the twist slowly when ready.

For the other side, either position both feet flat on the floor with your feet, knees, and thighs together, or put your left leg over the right. Take your right hand and place it on the outside of your left knee and press gently. Keep your right arm extended.

With your back straight, slowly begin turning to the left. Start the twist from the waist and then move your chest, shoulders, neck, and finally your eyes. Take your other arm (left) and put it around your back near your waist. Breathe in as you lengthen your spine and breathe out as you twist gently. Release the twist slowly when ready.

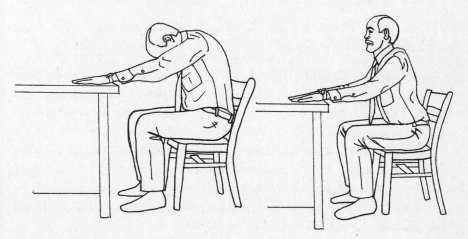

6. Cat Stretch. Your neck, shoulders, and entire spine will be stretched and lengthened; circulation to your spine will increase; respiration and digestion will improve; and your stomach muscles will be toned and tightened.

Make sure your chair is pushed away from your desktop so that you can sit on your chair and stretch both arms and hands straight out toward the desk. Place your fingers on the desktop or on your knees.

Next, lower your head as you arch your back up as you breathe out. On the next in-breath, raise your head and chest up while you curve and stretch your back in the other direction. Don't strain. Continue up and down, breathing in and out as you go. Rest for a few moments with your arms outstretched, and relax.

With your arms in the same position, begin looking over your right shoulder. Let your right arm stay stretched out as your left elbow bends a little. You will notice a nice back twist. Then slowly swing your torso back to the center, and look over your left shoulder. Let your arms and back move with you. Go back and forth a couple more times in a smooth manner and remember to keep breathing.

7. Seated Child's Pose. Although simple, this pose is packed full of benefits. It stretches your back, massages the organs of the abdomen, and releases the neck.

Begin breathing out as you slowly bend over so that the front of your body is resting on your lap. Your arms and hands can hang beside your legs and toward the floor.

Continue to take slow, even, and deep breaths as you let your head and neck hang comfortably forward.

8. Modified Shoulder Stand. You're going to have to get on the floor for this one. It's worth it. Your back will get a rest, the circulation in your legs will increase, and your energy will improve. If your work area doesn't have adequate wall space, try using a door, or the side of a file cabinet.

Sit on the floor about six inches from the wall. Your shoulder is facing the wall, your knees are bent with your rear end and feet on the floor. Slowly swing your legs and feet up so they rest on the wall and swing your back around so it's lying flat on the floor and perpendicular to the wall. Bend your knees slightly, especially if it is more comfortable.

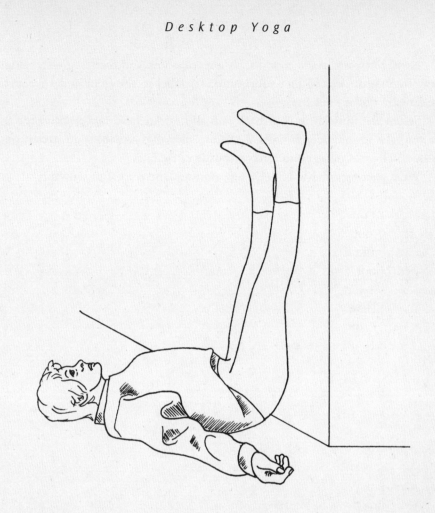

There you have it, your legs are in the air, your heels are resting against the wall, your knees are softly bent, and your back is flat on the floor. Now is a good time to practice your diaphragmatic breathing. You can even close your eyes. Give yourself time to get revived.

To get up, bend your knees and roll to the side, use your arms for support, and sit up.

9. Standing Back Stretch. This relaxing posture will relieve muscular tension while toning, stretching, lengthening, and massaging your back muscles.

Stand up first and treat yourself to a spontaneous stretch to your arms, back, and legs.

Next, rest your hands comfortably on your desk and then begin stepping away from your desk so that your spine is parallel to the floor and your feet are directly under your hips.

Soften the muscles in your back and allow your head and neck to relax. As you take several deep breaths, continue allowing your back to stretch on its own. There is no need to force or push yourself.

Walk your feet forward after a few minutes and return to standing.

eight

Legs and Feet

So much is expected from your feet and legs. They are required to walk, run, and jump. Sitting for long periods of time can impair the circulation to the legs, especially if you usually sit with your legs crossed. Not only that, work shoes are rarely designed with comfort in mind. It's no wonder we end up with weak ankles, flabby thighs, and varicose veins.

Fight back and try these leg and foot relievers. If possible, take off your shoes for these.

1. Knee Presses will tone and strengthen the muscles in your thighs.

Firmly press your knees and thighs together and hold for a few moments. Feel the tension. Then release your knees and let them separate. Take a few breaths and repeat once or twice.

2. Foot Rolls will improve circulation; strengthen and tone your feet, ankles, and legs; and keep them from getting stiff after sitting for a while.

Stretch your right leg out in front of you and begin moving your foot around in a big circle. Let your foot, ankle, and calf get in on the act. Are you still breathing? Now, circle your foot around in the other direction.

Next, point your toes forward and then back toward your head. Do this several times in a row.

Then, keep your leg straight and move the ball of your foot from side to side.

Stretch your toes.

Place your right foot back on the floor and raise your left leg and foot up and stretch it out in front of you.

Begin moving your left foot around in a big circle. Let your foot, ankle, and calf move freely.

Now, circle your foot around in the other direction. You're still breathing, right?

Next, point your toes forward and then back toward your head. Do this several times in a row.

Then, keep your leg straight and move the ball of your foot from side to side.

Stretch your toes.

Finally, place your foot back on the floor. Remember, it's bad for circulation to cross your legs.

Hint: The foot rolls described above can be done with both feet at the same time.

3. Heel Lifts will improve the circulation in your legs and feet, tone your calves, and bring flexibility to your ankles. Kick your shoes off if you can, and stretch your toes out.

Lift up both heels and press your toes into the floor. Hold for a few seconds, and then lower your heels. Repeat these movements several times.

4. Foot Rub. It's true. When your feet hurt, you hurt all over. So, why not do something about it? Kick your shoes off and give yourself a foot massage. Remember to rub your ankles, the top and bottom of your feet, and each toe. Try rubbing vigorously, softly, and pressing down with your thumbs and fingers. Even use your knuckles. Be creative and enjoy yourself.

5. Leg Lifts will tone your legs, increase hip flexibility, improve circulation, and strengthen your stomach and lower back.

Stand beside a steady chair with your left hand placed on the chair back to help your balance.

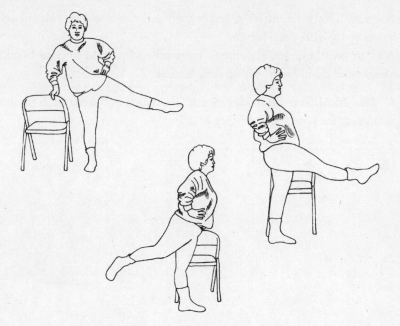

Forward Lift. Breathe in as you slowly lift your right leg up in front of you. Your knee can either be bent or straight. Breathe out as you lower your foot back to the floor. Breathe in again and raise, breathe out, and lower. Do this several more times. Practice coordinating the length of your breath to the leg movements.

Backward Lift. This time, breathe in while raising your leg up behind you as high as is comfortable. Breathe out as you lower. Repeat several times.

Side Lift. Now it's time to raise your leg up sideways. That's right, breathe in as it raises and breathe out as it lowers. Resist the urge to strain.

Next, stretch the left leg. Once again, place your right hand on the chair back for balance.

Forward Lift. Lift your left leg up in front of you as you breathe in fully. You may have to either increase or decrease your speed depending upon the length of your breath. Breathe out as you lower your foot back to the floor. Keep going for a few more rounds.

Backward Lift. Bring your leg up behind you as you breathe in and lower on the out-breath. Repeat several times.

Side Lift. This time, lift your left leg up and down to the side, matching the movements with your breath.

All this breathing and moving is extraordinarily good for you because it encourages the mind–body–breath connection.

6. The Modified Shoulder Stand described and illustrated in chapter 7 is also great for your legs and feet.

nine

Standing Poses

Sitting still all day is horrible on the back, and it hurts your circulation. Did you know that sitting is more strenuous than standing or lying down? It is.

Give yourself a break and stretch your legs and back from time to time. Take a walk, climb the stairs, and try these standing postures.

1. Foot Stompers. This is just like it sounds. Kick your shoes off and march around your work space. As you warm up, begin raising your knees higher and higher. Dance a jig, hop up and down, have fun. Let your breath be free. Stompers will reduce stress, and increase circulation to your feet, ankles, and legs. Your heart rate and respiration will increase.

2. Mountain Pose. This yoga standard will improve your posture, increase your awareness, and facilitate your physical and mental sense of balance and stability. The mountain pose will center your mind, strengthen your spirit, and stabilize your emotions. Use it to create a balanced feeling whenever you feel flustered or are about to climb the walls.

Take your shoes off and stretch your toes. Ahhh.

Stand with your feet placed about shoulder-width apart (an alternative is to stand with your big toes together with your heels placed a few inches apart so that the outsides of your feet are parallel to each other).

Shift your weight from side to side and back and forth. Stay in touch with the sensations in your feet.

Become still by evenly distributing your weight on both feet. Let there be equal pressure on your toes and heels. Feel your feet planting themselves firmly into the ground.

Turn your attention to your kneecaps. Begin raising them up by contracting the muscles in the front of your thighs. Let the awareness in your legs come alive.

Draw your attention up to your pelvis and discover its point of balance. Let your pelvic bones and pubic bone be aligned so that your low back doesn't curve and sway, or your stomach and hips lean forward.

Feel an opening and lengthening beginning to grow from your navel up through your breastbone. Notice the gentle massage of your breath.

Let your shoulders and arms relax as much as possible. Unclench your hands and soften your fingers.

Let your chin be parallel to the floor.

Pretend that there is a colorful ribbon pulling the top of your head gently up toward the sky.

Relax and let your breath move in and out of your lungs like ocean waves flowing back and forth on the sand.

3. Willow Tree. This pose will promote flexibility in the upper body, relieve stress, and improve circulation.

Stand up with your feet about shoulder width apart. Sway your entire body from side to side to include your shoulders, arms, hands, torso, hips, and knees. If you wish, imagine all your tiredness and troubles flowing out through your fingers and away from you. Enjoy the loose and free movements.

4. Hip Rolls. These movements will increase your range of motion, open the hips and pelvis, and improve the flexibility in your lower back.

Stand with your feet shoulder-width apart. Keep your knees slightly bent and take a few deep breaths.

Begin moving your hips as if you are doing the hula. Be sure to circle round in both directions. Let your knees move, too. See if you can make a figure eight with your hips.

5. Forward Fold. This wonderful posture will stretch and strengthen your arms, shoulders, and entire back; increase circulation to the spine, face and brain; and improve digestion.

Once again, stand with your feet at shoulder-width. Clasp your hands together behind your back.

Stretch your shoulders back and feel the opening around your heart and lungs. Notice the squeezing sensation near your shoulder blades. Breathe in as deeply as you can.

As you breathe out, slowly and carefully begin bending forward. Be sure to bend from the hinge in your hips and keep your back long and flat. It's better on your back not to use a curving motion.

Bend your torso as far forward as you comfortably can without feeling stress or strain to your back.

Let your head continue down and aim the crown of your head toward the floor.

Stretch your arms up behind you to feel the nice stretch to your back.

To come up, keep the bend in your knees and breathe in as you straighten up.

Tighten your buttocks and bend back slightly.

Repeat several more times.

6. Hero II (Warrior II). This pose will reward you with physical and mental stamina, strengthen your back and legs, and tone your arms and ankles. Your flexibility and balance will increase. It's great to practice when you would rather feel strong and stable instead of scattered.

Stand with your feet a comfortable distance apart (ideally your feet should be four to four and a half feet apart—you'll have to adjust your stance depending on your flexibility and your clothes).

Angle your left foot in about thirty degrees (it will look a little pigeon-

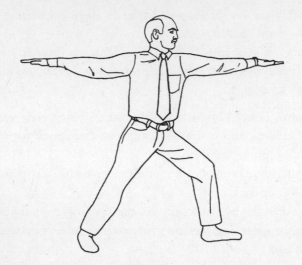

toed) and turn your right foot out to ninety degrees. Take time to line up the toe and heel of your right foot with the arch of your left foot.

Bend your right knee so that it's directly over your heel. This will form a right angle between your shin and the floor.

Be sure to keep your torso straight and raise your arms out to both sides until they are even with your shoulders. Look to the fingertips of your right hand and breathe evenly. Step your feet back to center.

Now it's time for the other side.

Place your right foot at about thirty degrees and turn your left foot out to ninety degrees. Once again, line up the toe and heel of your left foot with the arch of your right foot.

Bend your left knee so that it's directly over your heel to form a right angle between your shin and the floor.

Raise your arms out to both sides until they are even with your shoulders. Look to the fingertips of your left hand and breathe evenly.

Bring both feet back to center.

7. Downward-facing Dog with Chair. This one is great for relieving the stiffness in your upper back, shoulders, and legs. It will strengthen your arms and improve your posture.

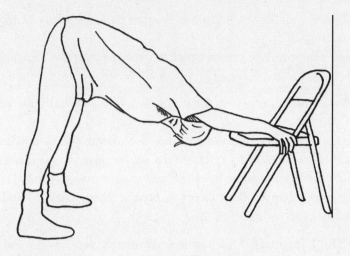

First, push a chair back securely against the wall with the chair seat facing you. Use a chair without wheels for this one.

Extend your arms straight down from your shoulders and grasp the chair seat with both of your hands. Your hands will be eight to twelve inches apart.

Straighten your arms while you walk your feet back about four steps behind you. Place your feet eight to twelve inches apart and parallel to one another.

Lift your rear end up toward the sky. Inhale and stretch your back away from your hands. Feel a long stretch from your hands through your arms and shoulders and then to your tailbone. Let the stretch extend from your tailbone down through your legs and into your heels. Hold this position for five or six breaths.

Walk your feet forward and stand back up.

8. Desk Pushups will strengthen and tone your arms and back, and improve your circulation and respiration.

Stand up and put your hands on the edge of your desk. Slowly straighten your arms and step back about three feet. Bring your feet together.

Your arms will be straight as you maintain a straight line from the top of your head down through your heels.

Exhale and bend your elbows slowly to lower your head and body toward the desk.

Straighten your elbows and push yourself back and away from the desk while breathing in.

Repeat this sequence several times in a row to improve your upper body strength.

9. Wall Squats are perfect for strengthening the back, thighs, calves, and abdomen.

Stand with your back against a wall or door. Begin sliding down until you are sitting on an imaginary chair. Make any necessary adjustments so that your thighs are horizontal to the floor and your shins are vertical. Hold this for thirty seconds or so. Don't forget to breathe. Raise back up and repeat a few more times.

10. Thigh Stretch. This posture will stretch your thighs and improve your flexibility.

Stand up and hold onto a bookshelf, filing cabinet, or wall for support.

Begin bending your right knee as you lift your right foot slowly up behind you and toward your buttocks. Straighten your knee to lower. Repeat several times.

As usual, it's time for the other side. Lift your left foot up toward your buttocks with a bend in the knee.

Breathe in as you raise and breathe out as you lower.

ten

Power Naps and Guided Relaxation

A yoga session is never complete unless time is spent relaxing at the
end. Doing so allows the benefits of all the postures to sink in and be
absorbed.

You will soon discover that a few minutes spent doing the following exercises, also known as "power napping," will do you a world of good. You
will actually discover the difference between muscular tension and relaxation. It's like taking a two-minute nap that feels like you have slept a full
two hours. Don't be misled, however; there's no substitute for a good night's
sleep.

If you can, put a Do Not Disturb sign on your office door and forward
your phone calls. (Being interrupted or startled is unpleasant and counterproductive.) Dim the lights and turn on some quiet, soothing music. Adjust your chair so that you can stretch your arms and legs straight out
in front of you. It's also better if you remove your shoes, necktie, and
glasses.

Here are several ways to help you get the full benefit from these experi-
ences.

1. Have someone softly and slowly read the instructions to you.

2. Familiarize yourself with the instructions and proceed on your own.

3. Make an audio recording to play back.

4. Follow the directions as you read through the instructions.

5. The ellipses(. . .)used throughout the following exercises indicate a brief pause.

The most important thing is to do it!

One to Ten

This is a short, three-to-six minute relaxation exercise that can be done either sitting in a chair or lying down. It is a good way to relax when time is limited or after you have become accustomed to going through a longer, more thorough progressive relaxation experience.

Begin by closing your eyes . . . and let the air in your lungs be released. . . . Take in a full, deep breath through your nose, allowing your lungs to fill up completely, letting the air go all the way in, and then sigh it out through an open mouth. Let all of the tiredness, tension, and negativity be released with your breath.

Take in another big deep breath . . . and sigh it out. Take your time . . . breathing in . . . and out . . . now, let your breath return to normal.

Next, you will slowly begin squeezing all the muscles throughout your body at the same time—your arms and legs, your torso and back, your shoulders and face. At the count of five, your body will feel half the way to being tense all over. By the count of ten, you will feel tension and tightness throughout your entire body. Then you will count backward from ten to one. As you do, you will slowly release the tension in your body. By the count of five, you will be half the way to feeling totally relaxed. At the count of one, your body will be relaxed completely. Then you will take in a nice, big breath, and then sigh it out.

As you sit or lie there, get a solid sense of your body as it is pressing firmly against the floor or chair . . . your awareness explores how your body is feeling right now, your legs . . . back . . . arms . . . and head. You are becoming acutely aware of how you are feeling in your physical body right now. Just become aware. . . .

Let's begin. One, just a little tension . . . two . . . add some more . . . three . . . four . . . five, you are halfway there, six . . . seven . . . eight . . . nine . . . and ten, you are all the way there now. Feel the contractions, and know it and experience it completely, so that you will be able to recognize muscular tension and tightness later on.

Nine, release a little bit . . . eight . . . let a little bit more go . . . seven . . . six . . . five . . . you are halfway there . . . four . . . three . . . two . . . one. Let all of the muscular tension and tiredness be dissolved and released. Let go totally. Experience fully the feeling of being completely relaxed and calm. . . . Let it soak in. . . . Learn to recognize the feeling of relaxation. . . .

If you still feel some muscular tension, you'll notice that you can relax even more if your mind gives your body permission to relax further. Let those spots relax now by mentally giving yourself permission to do so. . . . It's okay to relax. . . .

Take a nice big, deep breath and sigh it out, letting the air rush out through an open mouth. Let the air stay out of your body as long as comfortable and then take in another big, deep breath and sigh it out completely. Notice that you can relax more and more, each time you exhale. . . . Let your breath return to normal.

Notice how you feel . . . like you are sinking into the floor or chair. Let the floor or chair support and hold you, letting you feel safe and secure. Your body feels as if it's being supported completely and entirely. Every time you breathe out, you feel more and more relaxed, calm, and serene.

Draw your attention to your mind now. . . . Notice what's on your mind right now, what thoughts are going through. . . . Let your mind and thoughts become still so that you can begin to center in and concentrate more. . . . If your mind begins to wander, gently bring your attention back to this very moment or to your breath.

Now, notice how your emotional self is feeling right now. What kind of mood are you in? Try not to judge your mood, just notice and accept what you are naturally experiencing at this moment.

Each time you exhale, notice that you feel more and more settled and are feeling a sense of harmony and balance occurring within your body, mind, mood, and spirit. Feel a sense of balance within your body . . . mind . . . and emotions.

Whenever you are ready, you can begin to stretch and move, feeling refreshed and relaxed.

"One to Ten" is available on a tape called *Refreshing Journeys,* recorded by Julie Lusk. The tape has six delightful relaxation and guided imagery exercises on it. Call Whole Person Press at 1-800-247-6789 to order a copy.

Expanding and Contracting

This two-to-four minute power nap is a relaxation exercise that is best done lying on the floor. If this is impossible, it can also be done from your chair. It's a fantastic and very effective way to relax in a few moments.

Close your eyes and begin settling down into the floor or chair . . . let yourself sink into the surface as you become aware of your physical body.

All at once, expand by reaching out and tensing your arms and legs, open your eyes up wide, and stretch out your tongue. Expand your chest and stomach and hold it for several moments.

Relax all at once by letting your body go loose and soft. Take a few moments to feel the relief of letting the tightness and tension leave.

Now, contract and pull in. Pull your feet and legs in. Bend your elbows and make two fists. Compress your abdomen. Squint your eyes, purse your lips, and scrunch up your nose. Hold . . . and then let go.

Take a full, complete breath and fill up the lower part of your lungs so that your abdomen raises up. Open your mouth and let the air rush out.

Take in another full, deep breath and fill up the middle and upper portion of your lungs, feeling your rib cage expanding. . . . Open your mouth and let the air rush out.

Let your breathing return to normal . . . and each time you breathe out, let yourself relax more and more.

Let your mind scan your body; give your body mental permission to relax even further.

Allow your toes and feet to soften and relax . . . feel the softening spread throughout your calves as they become relaxed . . . your knees are now relaxed . . . and let it spread to your thighs . . . let your hips soften. . . .

Now your lower back is relaxing . . . mid-back . . . upper back . . . and shoulders are all letting go. Allow your upper arms to relax . . . your elbows . . . your forearms . . . your hands and your fingers. Everything's relaxing.

Going inside, your torso and the organs in your abdomen are relaxing completely. . . . And now your lungs. . . .

Feel your neck and throat relax, and all the muscles in your face as well. Your mouth . . . cheeks . . . nose . . . eyes . . . and forehead are relaxed.

The feeling of relaxation now spreads from the top of your head to the back of your head and all the way back down to your toes. Feel yourself become more and more relaxed. . . .

When ready, begin to stretch and move gently. Open your eyes, and you'll feel calm, relaxed, and rested.

Easy Does It

This is a different technique that will not require you to squeeze your muscles prior to relaxing them. Try this if you are especially tired or if you have physical conditions such as arthritis, fibromyalgia, or any other problem in tensing your muscles. Give yourself about five minutes for this one.

Let yourself sink comfortably into your chair. If possible, kick your shoes off and put your feet up.

Begin taking a few deep and full breaths as preparation for a relaxing experience. . . .

Slowly, breathe all the way in . . . and all the way out. . . . Each time you breathe out, begin releasing any tightness or tenseness you may have. Tightness may be in the form of physical tension, mental confusion, or emotional distress. . . . Just let it clear away, each time you exhale. . . .

Now, imagine that you are breathing in through your feet . . . and feel them soften and relax as you breathe out. Slow and easy.

Breathe in and let your awareness fill your legs . . . and slowly breathe out, noticing your calves . . . your knees . . . and your thighs. Every time you breathe out, release and let go.

Breathe in and wrap your awareness around your hips, feeling them soften as you breathe out . . . sinking and settling down. Slow and easy.

Breathe in as your attention floats to your back. . . . Feel the tension in your back dissolve, letting go more and more, each time you breathe out.

Breathe in and surround your shoulders with your awareness and feel them soften as you breathe out . . . releasing the tightness, the soreness, and the tension . . . soothing your shoulders with your slow and easy breath.

Breathe in and unclench your teeth . . . let your lips part slightly. As you continue breathing gently and softly, let your nose and cheeks smooth out . . . and your eyes and forehead soften.

Let this relaxed feeling begin flowing down around your shoulders and surrounding your arms and hands with peace and quiet.

Let your pores open up and breathe . . . feel yourself releasing and expanding.

As you relax deeper and deeper, the peacefulness reminds you of a quiet, personal sanctuary . . . an extremely comfortable and safe place where you feel surrounded with exactly what you need.

This is a special place where you can safely explore your very own inner thoughts and feelings . . . a place to feel protected and safe and understood . . . where you can spend some time getting to know the real you . . . the person you were meant to be . . . fully capable of finding answers to your questions . . . and feeling safe to be who you really are. Treat yourself to some time to explore this special feeling and space.

After a while, allow your attention to come back to your breath . . . feeling more wholesome and real.

And, whenever you are ready, begin to stretch your body, wiggle your fingers and toes . . . and open your eyes . . . feeling refreshed and renewed.

Very Short and Very Sweet

This exercise is based upon a simple breathing technique that is proven to clear your mind and freshen your spirit. While it may be difficult to stay focused at first, it gets easier and more effective with practice. Feel free to spend one to ten minutes on this experience.

Sit comfortably and begin clearing your mind. Allow yourself to forget about the past and let go of the future so you can stay focused upon each and every present moment.

Breathe in and silently say to yourself, "I am."

Breathe out and silently say, "calm and collected."

Breathe in and silently say, "I am."

Breathe out and silently say, "calm and collected."

Continue on for as long as you desire. As you practice, your mind will more than likely wander far and wide. Don't worry, this is very common. As soon as you notice that you've become distracted, simply let the distracting thought go and gently bring your attention back to your breath and your saying. The more you practice, the longer you will be able to stay focused. A bonus is that your ability to concentrate in general will improve in all sorts of situations and circumstances.

For variety, please feel free to substitute a different, positive saying that may have more appeal or meaning to you. For example, you may want to try "I am . . . healthy and happy," or "I am . . . strong and whole."

Seated Progressive Muscular Relaxation

This longer progressive relaxation experience is perfect for sitting in a chair. Allow fifteen to twenty minutes for the experience.

Close your eyes and begin feeling the sensation of relaxation. . . . Take a nice big breath, bringing your shoulders up toward your ears. Now, drop your shoulders down while releasing your breath. . . . Let's repeat, bring fresh air into your lungs, squeezing your shoulders up toward your ears, and hold. . . . Now let your shoulders drop down and relax as you release your breath. . . .

Hold your right arm straight out in front of you and make a tight fist with your thumb on the outside. Hold, tighter and tighter. One . . . two . . . three . . . four . . . five. . . . Drop your hand to your lap and relax.

This time, hold out your left arm, making a tight fist with your thumb on the outside. One . . . two . . . three . . . four . . . five. . . . Now, relax, let your arm relax completely, resting on your lap. . . .

Take time to hold both arms out and make a fist with your thumbs out; notice the tension in your wrist and at the back of your hands. One . . . two . . . three . . . four . . . five. . . . Relax. . . .

This time, hold your right arm straight out, bending your hand backward so your fingers point toward the ceiling. One . . . two . . . three . . . four . . . five. . . . Relax, allowing your arm to fall to your lap. . . .

Now hold your left arm straight out with your fingers pointing toward the ceiling. One . . . two . . . three . . . four . . . five. . . . Relax. . . . Notice the warm feeling in your arms. . . .

This time, hold out both arms, and tense both arms in the same manner. Feel the tension in the upper portion of your forearms. One . . . two . . . three . . . four . . . five. . . . Relax. . . .

Notice the feeling of relaxation in your arms. Warm and tingly. . . .

Now it's time to tense and relax your biceps. Bring the fingers of your right hand to your right shoulder and tense your biceps. One . . . two . . . three . . . four . . . five. . . . Relax, letting your arm fall to your lap. . . .

Next, bring the fingers of your left hand to your left shoulder, and hold. One . . . two . . . three . . . four . . . five. . . . Relax. . . .

Bring both hands to your shoulders and squeeze the biceps. Hold one . . . two . . . three . . . four . . . five. . . . Relax. . . .

Be aware of the feeling of relaxation in your arms. Warm, heavy, and comfortable. . . .

Allow your attention to focus on your legs. . . .

Draw your attention to the lower part of your thighs. Press your knees together so that the area of your legs above the knees are touching. One . . . two . . . three . . . four . . . five. . . . Relax. . . .

Hold your right leg straight out with your toes pointing forward. Squeeze your leg, one . . . two . . . three . . . four . . . five. . . . Relax, letting your foot fall to the floor. . . .

Now, hold your left leg straight out with your toes pointing forward, and squeeze. One . . . two . . . three . . . four . . . five. . . . Relax. . . .

This time, hold both legs straight out with your toes pointing forward. Notice the tension in your calf muscles. One . . . two . . . three . . . four . . . five. . . . Relax. . . .

Now shift your attention to below the kneecap. Hold your right leg straight out and point your toes toward your head. One . . . two . . . three . . . four . . . five. . . . Relax. . . .

This time, hold your left leg straight out and point your toes toward your head. One . . . two . . . three . . . four . . . five. . . . Relax. . . .

Hold both legs out in this way, noticing the area below the kneecap. One . . . two . . . three . . . four . . . five. . . . Relax. . . . You are feeling more and more at ease . . .

Notice that your legs and arms feel heavy . . . warm . . . and relaxed. Resolve to allow them to remain still and relaxed.

We are now going to relax the entire abdominal region. Draw in your abdominal muscles as much as you can. One . . . two . . . three . . . four . . . five. . . . Relax, feeling all of the knots inside letting go. . . .

Next, push your abdominal muscles outward as much as you can. One . . . two . . . three . . . four . . . five. . . . Relax. You're feeling more and more relaxed. . . .

Shift your attention to the chest area. Take in a deep breath and hold. One . . . two . . . three . . . four . . . five. . . . Let all of the air rush out, and relax. . . .

We are now going to concentrate on relaxing your neck. It's important to learn to relax this area since tension tends to accumulate there.

Tip your head directly to the right side, moving your right ear toward your right shoulder. Be careful not to strain one . . . two . . . three . . . four . . . five. . . . Let your head come back up to center. Let your head wobble until it comes to a comfortable resting position. . . .

Now let your left ear lower down toward your left shoulder. One . . . two . . . three . . . four . . . five. . . . Let your head return to center and let it wobble until comfortable. . . .

To relax the muscles in the front of your neck, bend your head forward and bring your chin toward your chest. One . . . two . . . three . . . four . . . five. . . . Relax and let your head wobble. . . .

Press your lips tightly together and hold, one . . . two . . . three . . . four . . . five. . . . Relax, letting your lips part slightly to relax your mouth. . . .

This time, bring your tongue upward and press it against the roof of your mouth. One . . . two . . . three . . . four . . . five. . . . Relax, letting your lips part slightly. . . .

To loosen up your jaw, open your mouth and move your jaw up and down and back and forth, working out all tension. . . . Relax. Let your lips part slightly. . . .

Wrinkle up your nose to tense the nose and cheeks. One . . . two . . . three . . . four . . . five. . . . Relax. . . .

Even though your eyes are closed, close your eyes tightly and feel the tension in your eyes and forehead. One . . . two . . . three . . . four . . . five. . . . Relax. . . .

Bring your attention to your forehead, frown, and lower your eyebrows downward. One . . . two . . . three . . . four . . . five. . . . Let go of all the tension and relax.

This time, draw your eyebrows upward. One . . . two . . . three . . . four . . . five. . . . Relax. . . .

It's now time to scan your entire body mentally. If you notice any remaining tension, give permission to that area to relax and let go. . . .

You are now very, very relaxed. . . . Take time to enjoy this delicious feeling. . . . Allowing this feeling to sink in all over. . . .

When you feel finished, start to picture the room you're in.

When you're able to picture the room, open your eyes and stretch.

Variations

If time doesn't permit you to do all of the above, it's okay to tense and relax each side separately without tensing both sides together. Another alternative is to tense the right and left sides at the same time. A different option is to relax a few areas at a time. You may stop counting to five after becoming accustomed to the length of time needed to feel the tension and the relaxation, and when you're comfortable with doing the exercise.

part two

Combinations and Special Sequences to Get You Through the Day

eleven

All Body Moves and Sequences

Who has time to do all of the Desktop Yoga movements? Certainly not anyone who has a job to do. Yet it is very important to fit a variety of stretches into your day—every day. Your body and your mind will reward you for your time and effort.

Begin building your daily routine by choosing the poses you enjoy the most. Be sure to choose movements from each section to create a balanced practice.

Here are a few sequences for your health and pleasure. Some of the components are new and some are arrangements of exercises that were previously described. Please feel free to design your own combinations, especially after you become more familiar with the poses and discover your personal favorites.

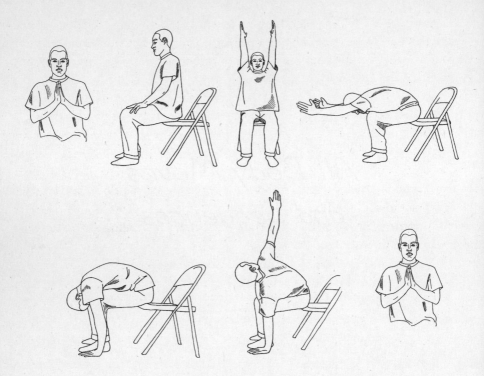

The Seated Sun Salute

This sequence is great to do when your time is limited and you want to cover a lot of stretches.

Move your chair out from your desk so you have lots of room.

Sit forward so your buttocks are on the seat of your chair and your thighs aren't. Take your shoes off.

Place both feet on the floor about hip-width apart. Feel your feet touching the floor. Let your weight be distributed equally upon both feet. Take some time to feel your toes, balls of your feet, heels, and both sides of your feet touching the ground. Stretch your toes.

Bring your fingers and palms together and place them in the center of your chest over your heart. Notice what this feels like and take several slow breaths.

Breathe out as you slowly lower your hands to the outside of your legs.

Breathe in as you slowly bring your arms up and over your head. Let your movements flow smoothly (stretches both sides of your body).

Breathe out as you begin hinging forward from the hips (keep your back straight) until your upper body is resting on your lap. Let your arms relax toward the floor with your arms on the outside of your legs near your feet (stretches the low back).

If you can, place your right palm flat on the floor next to the outside of your right foot. If you can't touch, just reach as far as is comfortable.

Breathing in, swing your left arm to the side and up until it points toward the ceiling. Look up to your hand.

Breathe out while you lower your left hand to the floor, so that your hand is near the outside of your left foot. If you can't reach the floor, just let your arm hang toward the floor.

Breathe in as you swing your right arm toward the ceiling as you look up. Experience the nice spinal twist.

Breathe out as you lower your right arm back down.

Breathe in as you stretch both arms out in front of you while raising them up over your head. Keep your back flat and move up from the hinge of your hips. This strengthens the lower back.

Breathe out and lower your hands back down in front of your chest with your palms touching.

Lower your hands to your lap, relax, and smile naturally.

The Seated Moon Salute

Scoot your chair out so there is lots of space in front of you as well as to your sides.

Sit firmly and squarely on the edge of your seat. Sit up tall and make certain that you are actually sitting on your sit bones rather than on your tailbone. Place your feet about twelve to fifteen inches apart.

Lengthen your spine by pressing your weight and attention down through your sit bones and up through the crown of your head. Notice the feeling of space that is being created between each of the spinal vertebrae.

Bend your elbows and gently press your hands together in front of your heart. Take some time to breathe in and out fully for several rounds. Doing this will help you feel centered and will calm you down.

Breathe out and slowly stretch your arms and hands out to your sides and level with your shoulders.

Breathe in and begin raising your hands and arms up over your head and finally interlace your fingers together. Point your index fingers toward the sky.

As always, practice coordinating your movements with your breathing.

Breathe out as you gently press your left foot and hip down while you are swaying your arms and upper body to the right.

Breathe in as you sway your arms and body back to the center.

Breathe out as you press your right foot and hip down while you are swaying your arms and upper body to the left.

Breathe in as you center your arms up overhead.

Breathe out as you separate your hands while bending your elbows. Lower your arms until your hands are level with your ears with your elbows stretched out wide open. Your palms are facing forward and you can feel a squeeze between your shoulder blades.

Breathe in and slowly stretch your arms out to both sides. Keep your arms level to your shoulders.

Exhale as you move into the seated triangle pose. Do this by smoothly lowering your right hand to the side of your right foot while you are raising your left arm toward the sky.

Inhale and move your body back to the center with your arms stretched out to both sides.

Exhale and lower your left hand to the side of your left foot while you're raising your right arm toward the sky.

Inhale and move your body back to the center with your arms out from your shoulders and to both sides.

Breathe out and bend your elbows. Keep the upper arms parallel to the floor. Bend at your elbows and point your fingers upward.

Breathe in and slowly raise your arms overhead and interlace your fingers together with your index fingers pointing straight up.

Breathe out as you press your right foot and hip gently down while you're swaying your arms and upper body to the left.

Breathe in as you sway your arms and body back to the center.

Breathe out as you press your left foot and hip down while you're swaying your arms and upper body to the right.

Breathe in as you center your arms up overhead.

Breathe out and lower your hands until they are in front of your heart and resting together, and take several more breaths.

Finally, lower your hands and let your breath return to normal.

Sequence to Calm Down

As you already know, it's easy to get bent out of shape at work. There are deadlines to meet, bosses to please, office politics to negotiate, coworkers to put up with, and work to get done. Instead of letting it get you down, use some of your Desktop Yoga for relief. Just a few minutes can make a world of difference in regaining your composure.

Three-Part-Breathing

Practice three-part breathing as a reminder to use your lungs fully and completely. Not only will it relax you, it will replenish your energy and sharpen your thinking.

Begin by releasing all the air from your lungs through your nose. Squeeze out even more air by compressing your abdominal muscles.

Slowly and smoothly, begin breathing in through your nose. Let the air go in so deeply that you feel an expansion in the belly area. As more air flows in, your entire rib cage (front, back, and sides) expands. Finally allow the air to fill the collarbone area.

Let all the air be released slowly through your nose as you empty your lungs from the top to the bottom.

Continue three-part breathing for as long as you comfortably can. It's important that you don't rush or forcefully push the air in or out. Bring your awareness back to your breath each time your attention wanders away.

Willow Tree

Stand up tall with your feet about shoulder-width apart. Begin swaying your shoulders, arms, hands, torso, hips, and knees from side to side. As you sway back and forth, imagine all your tiredness and troubles flowing out through your fingers and away from you. Enjoy the loose and free movements.

Heart Warmer

Still standing, place both your hands over your heart area and feel for the beat of your heart. Take your time. Feel free to close your eyes to tune out distractions, and breathe naturally for several minutes.

On an in-breath, slowly sweep your arms out to the sides and in line with your shoulders. As you exhale, move your arms back in and fold your hands over your heart.

As you practice, see if you can synchronize your arm movements to coincide with the rate and rhythm of your breath. Repeat these movements five or so times.

Forward Fold

While standing, adjust your feet so they are shoulder-width apart. With your arms straight, clasp your hands together behind your back.

Stretch your shoulders back so that you are squeezing your shoulder blades toward each other. Feel the opening around your heart and lungs. Breathe in as deeply as you can.

Breathing out, slowly and carefully begin bending forward as far as possible without feeling stress or strain to your back. Be sure to bend from the hinge in your hips and keep your back long and flat. It's far better on your back not to use a curving motion.

Let your head continue forward, and aim the crown of your head toward the floor.

Stretch your arms and clasped hands up behind you to feel the nice stretch to your back.

To come up, breathe in as you straighten up while keeping a slight bend in your knees.

Continue the stretch by tightening your buttocks, and bend back a bit.

Repeat several more times. Remember to breathe out as you bend forward and breathe in as you straighten back up.

Hip Rolls

Stand with your feet shoulder-width apart with a slight bend to your knees. Take a few deep breaths.

Begin moving your hips in large circles. First circle around to the right for several times, and then circle around to the left. Let your knees move with you. After a while, see if you can make a figure eight with your hips.

Big Mouth

Release the tension in your mouth and jaw by opening and closing your mouth over and over. Then quickly move your jaw sideways to the right and left. Next, mix up and down movements with sideways ones. People with TMJ (Temporomandibular Joint Syndrome) should not do the movements to the sides.

Improvise

Let your body move you. Listen to it and follow it where it wants to take you. Of course, you may practice some of the Desktop Yoga moves you have already learned, or make up movements of your own.

Finishing Breath

Sit back down and give yourself a final stretch. Uncross your legs and place both of your feet flat on the floor (remember to use a footrest or thick book if your feet don't reach). Shift your back around so that it can maintain a balanced S-shaped curve.

Close your eyes while saying silently, "I am," and breathe out while saying "calm." Keep going until you really do feel calm. Remember to return your attention to your breath whenever your mind wanders.

Practical Measures

While Desktop Yoga has a lot to offer, don't forget to take a walk, lay off caffeine, and, whenever possible, avoid unpleasant situations and people.

Sequence to Get Energized

It's a wonderful thing to have ample energy to get your work done and enough left over for your private life. Unfortunately, it seems much more common to feel tired and rundown.

Try this sequence to bring yourself back to life.

Ujjayi Breathing

This is a powerful technique that will help build up your endurance and stamina while also improving your ability to concentrate.

Ujjayi breathing is done by making a slight constriction in the throat (glottis) during inhalation and exhalation.

Inhale and exhale with your mouth open while whispering "haaa." Notice the open feeling in your throat. Next, close your mouth and continue breathing fully while maintaining that open feeling in your throat.

Reclaim your energy by taking five to ten Ujjayi breaths in a row. Let your breath be as deep and slow as is comfortable for you.

Energy Stretch

This energizer can be done on your feet or sitting down. If you are sitting, place both feet flat on the floor and let your arms hang to your sides.

As you breathe in a slow Ujjayi breath, begin raising your arms straight out in front of you until they are shoulder height. Continue to breathe in; bring your arms out to both sides, and then raise them over your head.

Breathe out a slow Ujjayi breath as you lower your arms back down to your sides. Continue on for five to ten deep, diaphragmatic breaths.

The trick here is to raise your arms during the time it takes to take a breath in and to lower your arms during the time it takes to breathe out. Practice makes perfect.

Chest Expander

While either standing or sitting, clasp your hands together behind you with your arms straight down.

Raise your clasped hands and arms up behind you and squeeze your shoulder blades together.

Take in five to ten Ujjayi breaths.

Lower your arms and wiggle your arms and shoulders about.

Pattie, Pat Pat

Fold your hands into gentle fists with your thumbs on the outside. Open palms also work. Try both hand positions and decide for yourself which works best for you.

Begin patting gently all over the top of your head, face, and neck. Move down to your shoulders and arms.

Begin tapping the area near your tailbone and low back. Come around and continue tapping from your belly to your chest and back up to your shoulders.

Repeat the tapping of your back, belly, torso, and shoulders.

Start patting your hips, thighs, calves, and shins. Take your shoes off and pat the bottoms of your feet, too.

Finishing Breath

While sitting down, give yourself a final stretch. Uncross your legs and place both feet flat on the floor (remember to use a footrest if your feet don't reach). Align your back so that it maintains a balanced S-shaped curve.

Breathe in and say, "I am" and breathe out while saying "energized and strong." Keep repeating until your energy level improves. Remember to bring your attention back to your breath whenever it wanders.

Practical Measures

When feeling tired, don't forget to go outside and get some fresh air. And remember, there's nothing better than getting eight hours of sleep.

Sequence to Boost Creativity

Being creative is fabulous. This is especially true when there are problems to solve or something to make. Much of Desktop Yoga will automatically get your creative juices flowing because it slows you down long enough to let you actually think something out, nourish your brain by improving circulation, and keep stress from becoming unbearable.

Alternate Nostril Breathing

This soothes the nerves and stimulates the functioning of the entire brain. Creativity demands the capacity to be imaginative as well as to be realistic. Alternate nostril breathing encourages your ability to do both.

First, fold your pointer and middle fingers toward the palm of your right hand. Gently place your thumb against your right nostril and breathe out from your left nostril. Ujjayi breathing is highly suggested.

Next, breathe in through the left side and close the left nostril with your ring and pinky fingers. At the same time, release your thumb from the right nostril to release the air. Breathe in that same side and then gently press your thumb against the right nostril, release the ring and pinky fingers, and send the air out the left side. This completes one round.

Continue switching sides for several more rounds. Sixteen rounds is ideal. (Alternate Nostril Breathing is illustrated on page 15.)

Infinity Stretches

These delightful stretches foster flexibility and bring a sense of the infinite into your world. All that is needed is to trace the infinity symbol with different parts of your body. The infinity symbol is shaped like a sideways figure eight. While you're at it, imagine infinite possibilities coming to you as you practice. Let's begin with the hips and continue up the body.

Hips

Stand up and trace a sideways figure eight with your hips. Let your knees and hips sway and enjoy the movement. Do this five to ten times and then reverse the direction.

Arms and Hands

Clasp your hands together and stretch your arms straight out in front of you, level with your shoulders. Draw a very large infinity symbol in front of you. Do this five to ten times, and then reverse the direction.

Neck

Lower your shoulders and relax them. There's no need for unnecessary tension. Begin making the infinity symbol slowly and smoothly with your nose. See if you can do it just as smoothly in the opposite direction. Do each side five to ten times. Imagine your creativity stretching infinitely.

Eyes

Softly move your eyes in the shape of the infinity symbol as smoothly as you are able. Close your eyes and rest them. Open them back up and move them in the opposite direction. Close your eyes again and rest along with some full and complete breaths.

Seated Forward Fold

This will bring greater circulation to your brain, which will help you think more clearly and let your imagination soar.

Push your chair a little way out from your workstation and sit on the edge of your seat.

Place your feet flat on the floor and about eight to twelve inches apart. Creatively stretch your arms in all directions. Finally, let them rest at your sides and take a couple of nice, deep, smooth breaths.

Now, as you exhale, begin folding forward from your hips so that your upper body rests on your lap. Continue to breathe long, full breaths. Let your head hang down with your arms falling gently toward the floor. After you've had enough, breathe in as you sit back up.

Repeat the forward fold again. Refreshing your brain with more blood is extremely helpful. (This is illustrated as part of the Seated Sun Salute on page 72.)

Shoulder Wings

Rest your right hand on your right shoulder and your left hand on your left shoulder. Begin slowly and evenly flapping your arms as if they are wings. Increase the tempo and let your imagination take flight. (This is illustrated on page 26.)

Improvise

Stretch yourself out in all sorts of new and unusual directions. Have fun and remember to breathe.

Finishing Breath

Sit down, uncross your legs, and place both feet flat on the floor (remember to use a footrest if your feet don't reach). Shift your pelvis and spine into place so that it forms its normal S-shaped curve.

Breathe in and say, "I am," and breathe out while saying, "creative and imaginative." As always, bring your attention back to your breath whenever it wanders.

Sequence to Reduce Anger and Frustration

Foot Stompers

Kick your shoes off and march around your work space. As you warm up, begin raising your knees higher and higher. Really move. Dance a jig, hop up and down, have fun. Let your breath be free.

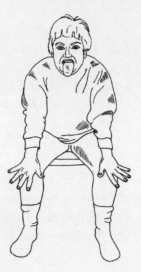

Lion Pose

This pose really releases frustrations as it brings a fresh supply of blood to your eyes, sinuses, and complexion. It's also good for your throat and voice box.

Sit with both your feet flat on the floor and place your hands on your knees. Now, take a big deep breath and let the air rush out as you bug out your eyes, stick your tongue way out, and stretch out your fingers. You'll notice a refreshing tingling feeling in your face, which is thought to work like a natural face-lift. It's a great emotional release.

Heart Opener

Make your hands into fists and begin to tap them all along your heart and chest.

Continue tapping your shoulders and then move the motions all over your body.

When you are warmed up, pound a bit harder and faster.

Breathwork

One of the last things you'll feel like doing when you are mad is sitting down and breathing. However, doing so works miracles and will help you release the anger and frustrations from your system. Try the releasing breath and cooling breath exercises to see which one works best for you.

Releasing Breath

Breathe in through your nose and forcefully breathe out through your mouth. This is even more effective if you compress your abdominal muscles on the out-breath. Imagine your anxious feelings being sent out each time you breathe out. Breathe in and out in this manner for several minutes.

Cooling Breath

Roll the sides of your tongue to form a small opening with your lips and tongue. Breathe in as if you are drinking cool refreshing water through a straw. And then slowly and evenly breathe the warm air out through your nose. Continue on until you have cooled down.

Finishing Breath

Sit down, uncross your legs, and place both feet flat on the floor. Align your pelvis, back, and neck into its normal S-shaped curve.

Breathe in and say "I release," and breathe out while saying "anger and frustration." As usual, bring your attention back to your breath whenever it wanders.

twelve

Yoga on the Go

More than ever, yoga is needed when traveling. While traveling can be fun, exciting, and productive, it can also pile on the pressure. Hectic schedules, strange places, unfamiliar food, jet lag, and inadequate sleep can really throw you off balance.

Desktop Yoga can definitely help you cope with all these potentially irritating changes. Unfortunately, it's too easy to forget how helpful and comforting yoga can be when in a new place and away from your normal routine. Luckily, yoga can be done anywhere and without special clothes or fancy equipment. The problem of locating a gym is eliminated.

By Car

Getting lost, being stuck in traffic, and running late are only a few hassles of car travel. How about riding with someone that drives you crazy? And why does it always seem that road work is in the way whenever you are in a hurry?

Driving long distances can be boring as well as hard on your back, legs, and neck. This often reduces the effectiveness of your circulatory and cardio-vascular systems.

Here are a few simple tricks to take the wear and tear out of car travel.

—Make sure that your car is in good working order. Take the extra time and spend whatever it takes to keep your car in good repair. It will lessen your worries, since there is nothing worse than breaking down.

—Create a healthy atmosphere. A blaring radio can really be nerve-wracking. Consider relaxing music or turning the volume down or off for a pleasant change. Buying or borrowing books on tape is entertaining and often educational.

—Don't smoke, especially in a closed-up car. It smells bad and pollutes the air. If you must smoke, consider stopping for a break, so you can also stretch your legs.

—Cut down on distractions. It's hard enough to deal with traffic without having to eat a sandwich or keep from spilling a drink. It won't kill you to stop long enough to eat, and your food will be easier to digest.

—Give yourself plenty of time. Rushing and worrying about being late are stresses that can be avoided.

—Prepare for the weather. Snow tires, chains, and working windshield wipers are worth the extra trouble and expense.

—Try to observe the speed limit.

—Don't drive on an empty tank.

—Pack a map in case you get lost or need additional directions.

—Carry a cellular phone or CB radio for emergencies. For safety's sake, please remember to pull off the road to make your phone call.

—Stop and stretch your legs every now and then. The few extra minutes may save your life.

—Breathe.

—Keep your head, neck, and back in proper alignment as much as possible. As you know, most car seats leave much to be desired. At the very least, extend and lengthen your neck upward, keep your chin parallel to the ground, and position your ears so they are above your shoulders. In other words, don't crane your neck forward or slouch.

—Practice yoga on the go at stoplights and when stuck in traffic.

By Plane

Air travel can be full of surprises, both nice and not so nice. Let's face it: the food is often bad, the air is stuffy, and the seats are cramped and uncomfortable. Bad weather causes delays, connections are poor, and getting around airports is often confusing. Anything you can do to prevent problems is important. Here are some suggestions:

—Get to the airport well in advance of your departure. Allow enough time for traffic delays, parking, security checks, and long lines.

—Drink plenty of water to keep yourself hydrated. At least eight to sixteen ounces every hour ought to do it. If you don't get enough water, you are likely to suffer from a dry mouth; racing pulse; dry skin, hair, and nails; constipation; infrequent urination; and the inability to sweat upon exertion. Unfortunately, alcohol and caffeinated drinks (cola, coffee, tea) increase the problem of dehydration.

—Pack a healthy snack or meal.

—Order ahead from the special menu selections. Low-fat, vegetarian, or low-sodium are some of the choices that are often easily available. Just call your travel agent or carrier in advance.

—Bring a Walkman along to listen to music you enjoy. Listening to a guided meditation tape is relaxing and you'll arrive at your destination feeling refreshed. Consider wearing the headphones, whether or not they are plugged in. Doing so may cut down on noise and discourage your seatmate from talking your ear off.

—Use an inflatable neck pillow to help you rest or sleep more comfortably.

—Watch out for jet lag when having to change time zones. In addition to practicing the other helpful hints for air travel, begin the process of resetting your biorhythms by assuming the schedule of the new time zone right away by sleeping, eating, and going about your normal activities in line with your destination. As soon as possible, get out into the early morning light for at least thirty minutes. Set your watch and alarm clock to the new time.

—Pack lightly. Not only will smaller bags be easier to carry, it's possible to avoid having to check your baggage. If you check your baggage, remember to carry your medicine and other valuables with you on the airplane.

—Try Sea-Bands if you get airsick. They are elastic bracelets that have a button which presses on a specific acupressure point located on the wrist to control nausea. They are available in most airport gift shops and in marine stores.

Yoga on the Go

Many Desktop Yoga stretches can be done in a car or on an airplane, so use your imagination and don't be shy. Here is a sequence to try when you are fresh out of ideas.

Neck Stretches

Let your right ear drop slowly to your right shoulder. Then, slowly and smoothly roll your head forward and to the left. Don't go beyond a semicircle. Next, move your head from the left over to the right.

Repeat these semicircles several times and remember to breathe. This will relieve the tension in your neck and upper back.

Neck Flex

Clasp your hands behind your head and slowly twist your head, neck, and elbows gently to the right. Look at your right elbow and take a few breaths.

Slide your head, neck, and arms back to the center and then toward the left.

Only move as far as you comfortably can. Gaze at your left elbow as you breathe evenly and smoothly. Go ahead and repeat these movements several times.

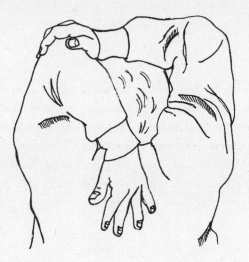

Elbow Up

This time, point your right elbow toward the sky with your arm and hand moving down toward the middle of your back. Place your left hand on your extended elbow and gently move it toward the center. Hold for a few breaths as you notice the wonderful stretch to your right shoulder.

Bring both arms down to your sides and wiggle your arms and shoulders around in all directions.

Now, position your left elbow straight up with your left arm and hand going down your back. Put your right hand on your left elbow, take a breath, and gently tug to the right. Apply just enough pressure so that you feel a nice stretch to your left shoulder.

Lower your arms and wiggle them around some more.

Shoulder Shrugs

Let your arms and shoulders relax at your sides. Stretch both shoulders up toward your ears while you breathe in through your nose.

Breathe out through your mouth as you let your shoulders drop back down. Really let go.

It's fine to repeat this a few more times. This releases frustrations as well as shoulder tension.

Shoulder Rolls

Sit forward and bring both shoulders up toward your ears, move them backward, feeling a squeeze between your shoulder blades, then move them all the way down and then toward the front. Repeat these circular movements while letting your arms and hands relax. Remember to breathe.

And now for the other direction, start with your shoulders as low as they go. Next move them forward, up, and to the back. This is done smoothly, evenly, and gently, just like your breathing.

Bridge Work

Softly pinch the bridge of your nose and massage the area between your eyebrows.

Rub and smooth out your forehead with your fingers and make soft circles at the temples. Remember to breathe.

Ear Rub

Use both of your hands to rub and massage your ears. This will stimulate the nerve endings that are located on the surface of your ears.

Surround your ears with your fingers by making a "V" with your pointer and middle fingers. Rub your fingers up and down, pressing firmly. Remember to unclench your teeth.

Big Mouth

Lots of people hold tension in the area surrounding the jaw. One way to help avoid this is to open and close your mouth quickly over and over. Move your jaw all around.

Palming

Resting your eyes from time to time can make your trip more enjoyable. Obviously, this makes more sense if you are flying or are an automobile passenger.

Rub your hands rapidly together with your palms and fingers touching. Keep rubbing until you feel some heat and energy being generated. Cup your hands and gently place them over your closed eyes. Let the warmth and darkness soothe your eyes. Take several long and easy breaths as you imagine the tiredness being released with your out-breath, and energy and vitality returning with your in-breath. Keep your shoulders down and relaxed.

Wrist Rolls

Let your arms fall to your sides or rest on your lap. Begin circling your wrists and hands round and round. First circle around one way, and then in the opposite direction. This is designed to improve your circulation and flexibility.

Hand Rub

Rub and massage one hand with the other. Remember to rub your wrist, palm, and each finger. As always, repeat on the other side.

Cat Stretch

Extend your arms and hands out and stretch your fingers and claws. Follow this by making fists. Finally, place your open hands on your knees.

Next, lower your head as you arch your back up and round it forward. Exhale. As you inhale, raise your head and chest up while you curve your back in the other direction. Don't overstretch. Continue moving back and forth, breathing in and out as you go. Rest for a few moments with your arms outstretched, and relax.

With your hands on your knees, begin looking over your right shoulder. Let your right arm stay stretched out as your left elbow bends a little. You will notice a nice spinal twist. Then slowly swing your torso back to the center, and look over your left shoulder. Let your arms and back move with you. Go back and forth a couple more times in a smooth manner and remember to keep breathing.

Knee Presses

Firmly press your knees and thighs together and hold for a few moments. Feel the tension. Then release your knees and let them separate from each other. Take a few breaths and repeat at least two or three more times.

Foot Moves

Stretch your right leg out in front of you and begin moving your foot around in a big circle. Let your foot, ankle, and calf get in on the action. Are you still breathing? Now, circle your foot around in the other direction.

Next, point your toes forward and then back toward your head. Do this several times in a row.

Then, keep your leg extended and move the ball of your foot from side to side.

Stretch your toes. Spread them apart and then make "fists."

Place your right foot back down and raise your left leg and foot up and stretch it out in front of you.

Begin moving your left foot around in a big circle. Let your foot, ankle, and calf move freely.

Now, circle your foot around in the other direction. You're still breathing, right?

Next, point your toes forward and then back toward your head. Do this several times in a row.

Then, keep your foot off the floor and move the ball of your foot from side to side.

Stretch your toes.

Finally, place your foot back down. Remember, it's bad for circulation to cross your legs.

Hint: To save time, the above can also be done with both feet at the same time.

Heel Lifts

If possible, take your shoes off and stretch your toes out.

Raise your heels and press your toes into the floor. Hold for a few seconds and then lower your heels.

This time, press your heels into the floor and raise your toes. Hold for a short while, and then lower.

Repeat these movements several times to improve the circulation in your legs and feet, tone your calves, and bring flexibility to your ankles.

Have a save and enjoyable trip.

part three

Replacing Worksite Worseness with Wellness

thirteen

Overdoing It:
Repetitive Strain Injuries

*I*t's becoming more and more difficult to escape from the information age of computers, faxes, E-mail, and the internet. It seems like you can't do anything, go anyplace, or work anywhere without coming in contact with these things. Fortunately, these tools have brought many blessings and advantages to our culture. However, spending hour after hour using your computer keyboard and mouse creates strain throughout your entire system. If you're not careful, it will eventually take its toll on your eyes, hands, wrists, neck, and shoulders. And if that's not enough, sitting still all day fosters poor circulation, is harmful to your back, can stiffen your skeleton, and will cause you to lose your energy and productivity.

According to the United States Bureau of Labor Statistics, over 60 percent of all workplace-related injuries can be attributed to cumulative stress injuries (repetitive strain injuries). These terms refer to a variety of syndromes that can affect the wrists, hands, shoulders, and neck that result from the damage done to tendons, nerves, muscles, or other soft tissues through overuse. Not only do computer users have to worry about these problems, people working on assembly lines and as seamstresses have had to be careful for years.

Types of Repetitive Strain Injuries

One of the most common repetitive motion injuries in computer users is **carpal tunnel syndrome** which is caused by compression of the median nerve in the wrist. The carpal tunnel is located at the base of the palm by the wrist. The top of the "tunnel" is covered by a strong band of connective tissue (ligament) and the sides and bottom are formed by wrist bones. The median nerve and nine tendons go from the forearm through the wrist into your hand through the tunnel. The median nerve provides sensations or feeling in the hand and fingers, and the tendons enable you to bend and move your fingers. Each tendon is covered by the synovium which is a lubricating membrane.

Carpal tunnel syndrome occurs when the median nerve is pressed against the ligament. This can happen when this area becomes compressed, inflamed, or swollen. Sometimes, the lubricating linings around the tendons thicken because of repetitive or too forceful hand movements. If the swelling is bad enough, it may result in pain, weakness, numbness, tingling, or a burning sensation in the wrist, palm, or fingers. Don't jump to conclusions however, have your thyroid checked since a hypothyroid condition sometimes presents itself as carpal tunnel pain.

Tendinitis occurs when tendons become inflamed and sore. It can occur in the shoulders, forearm, or hand. Acute tendinitis can be present following excessive overuse, whereas chronic tendinitis results from repetitive wear and tear due to age or from a degenerative disease.

Tenosynovitis is the swelling of the tendon and the sheath that covers it. Symptoms may involve swelling, tenderness, and pain in your hand or arm.

DeQuervain's disease is a particular form of tenosynovitis that can be especially troublesome for computer users. It causes acute pain where the thumb and wrist are joined. Specifically, irritation and swelling is present in the sheath or tunnel which surrounds the thumb tendons as they travel from the wrist to the thumb. The most common symptoms are felt as pain upon grasping or pinching and tenderness over the tunnel. The pain gets worse if your hand is shaped into a fist with the thumb tucked in and bent toward the little finger.

Symptoms of Repetitive Strain Injuries

Repetitive motion injuries can occur from overuse when highly repetitive movements are done with speed and force. Injury is also likely when awkward movements or a strange body position has to be held over time. Symptoms may involve:

—Tingling, pain, weakness, or numbness is felt in one or both of the hands. With carpal tunnel syndrome, one or two fingers are usually affected first, and it is often noticed in one hand more than the other. These sensations tend to be more common at night.

—Decreased feeling in your thumb, index, and long finger.

—Aching, burning, or painful sensations in the entire arm may be felt.

—Discomfort and pain is experienced from prolonged gripping (like a steering wheel, tool, or computer mouse).

—Clumsiness in handling things, such as a telephone or drinking glass, is noticed.

How to Prevent Repetitive Strain Injuries

Don't set yourself up for trauma trouble by going overboard in your work or leisure life. Avoid using repetition, poor position, and unnecessary force over an extended time to prevent repetitive motion injuries.

Repetition

Don't repeat the same motion in the same manner for long periods of time. Doing so will make you more likely to overuse your muscles and create physical stress. Take breaks and remember to stretch throughout the day.

Position

Holding your hands, wrists, and arms in an awkward position will put harmful pressure on your muscles, nerves, and tendons. Make an effort to improve your posture and alignment by adjusting your workstation and body position as described in chapter 3.

Force

Using too much pressure to perform a job or activity puts your muscles, nerves, and tendons at greater risk as well. Practicing the principles of yoga will help you remember to apply the correct amount of energy necessary to complete each task or movement.

Time

Another setup for trouble is having to repeat the same movements over and over again by the day, month, or year without sufficient rest. Once again, vary your workload to avoid having to spend too much time on one project and give yourself a sufficient rest period to recover from long periods of doing repetitive movements.

Traditional Treatments for Repetitive Strain Injuries

Early treatment for carpal tunnel syndrome, tendinitis, and tenosynovitis is a must. Traditionally, mild cases can be treated with rest to allow the swelling to shrink. Limiting or avoiding the activities that caused the symptoms is almost always needed. A brace or splint is sometimes recommended to help the affected area rest. Some people feel relief from cold treatments applied to the painful area while others prefer hot. Try both to see what is best for you. Nonsteroidal anti-inflammatory medications can be prescribed to reduce further the swollen membranes. In some instances, steroid injections may be needed to solve more severe cases. Those who do not respond to nonsurgical treatment may need outpatient surgery.

Complementary Treatments

Advocates of complementary medicine recommend a variety of nontraditional treatment modalities. Diet, nutritional therapy, aromatherapy, herbs, and homeopathy are a few options to consider. If you decide to go this route, be wise and choose a qualified practitioner that is knowledgeable about your problem. Ask about their training, experience, and certification. Avoid people who have solutions that are too good to be true or claim they can cure whatever ails you.

Diet and Nutritional Therapy

People with carpal tunnel syndrome often have a large vitamin B6 (pyridoxine) deficiency. Some think that this may cause a pyridoxine-responsive neuropathy (nerve disorder). Therefore, treatment with vitamin B6 may relieve symptoms. One place to start is to avoid foods that deplete vitamin B6. These include sugars, caffeine, processed grains, and corn. Choose a whole food diet and limit protein. Focus on whole grains, seeds, nuts, soybeans, fresh salmon, brewer's yeast, molasses, liver, wheat bran and germ, and cod.

Aromatherapy

Essential oils that have been extracted from herbs and plants are being used to treat a variety of medical conditions. Ones that reduce inflammation are recommended for repetitive strain injuries. Depending upon the particular oil, these substances can be inhaled or applied externally. Since the properties of essential oils are powerful, it is important to consult a reference guide or qualified professional for specific instructions in using aromatherapy.

Herbs

This branch of complementary medicine is also called botanical medicine, phytotherapy, or phytomedicine. It refers to using a plant or a portion of a plant (stem, leaves, root, etc.) for medicinal purposes. Whole herbs, teas, pills, extracts, tinctures, essential oils, salves, balms, and ointments can be used depending upon the herb and condition being treated. Anti-inflammatory herbs can be of benefit to repetitive strain injuries.

Homeopathy

Homeopathic preparations use extremely minute doses which are made from dilutions of natural substances such as plants, minerals, or animals. Used around the world, homeopathy is based on the principle that "like cures like." Homeopathic treatment for repetitive motion syndrome tends to be constitutional in nature and is therefore normally long-term, but usually successful.

Other Options

In addition, osteopathy, acupressure, applied kinesiology, chiropractic, craniosacral therapy, light therapy, naturopathic medicine, orthomolecular medicine, reconstructive therapy, and bodywork (acupressure, Feldenkrais, Hellerwork, Rolfing) may also be effective when provided by a qualified health professional.

Desktop Yoga Solutions

Luckily, you now have specific and helpful Desktop Yoga stretches, movements, and exercises to perform to prevent the development of major medical, emotional, or mental problems. Just knowing about these things, however, will never take the place of actually doing them. Somehow, you must find a way to slip in a neck roll, schedule a back stretch, and take time for a walk in the fresh air.

Not only is it beneficial to do the neck and shoulder exercises listed in chapter 4, but the shoulder stretches and back movements are equally important. Here are a few more stretches to do on a regular basis to improve circulation and relieve the stress and strain.

Hand Squeeze and Stretch

First, shape your hands into fists and rotate them from the wrist in one direction fifteen times. Stretch your fingers apart and continue to rotate your wrists. Change directions and repeat the rotations using both hand positions.

Thumb Stretch

Spread your fingers apart and gently pull your thumb back with your other hand. Hold this position while taking three slow breaths. Next, fold your thumb toward the palm of your hand and hold for three more breaths. Repeat these movements for up to five times and then stretch the other thumb and hand.

In short, repetitive strain injuries are nothing to fool around with. Take positive action to prevent problems. It's very important to get a proper diagnosis, sound recommendations, and early treatment from qualified professionals.

part four

A Better Way

Creating a Life—
Not a Lifestyle

*E*ach and every one of us has established a personal lifestyle—it may be one that's considered "desirable" or perhaps "undesirable" by somebody else's standards—but nevertheless, we all have a lifestyle. Furthermore, today's society has a way of constantly reminding us about our mistakes and problematic habits. As you know, it is almost impossible to pick up a newspaper, watch television, read a magazine, or go to a seminar where stress management and living a healthy lifestyle isn't at least mentioned.

Millions of us have poured time, money, and effort into creating a lifestyle. A lifestyle is meant to support living. However, how many of us have let our lifestyle get in the way of fruitful and meaningful living? Lifestyles can get in the way when they detract from our health and happiness and when they aren't genuine and authentic. For example, people get into trouble when they always put an overly ambitious exercise schedule in front of relationships with family and friends. But, continually placing family and friends over everything else can be just as bad. Living as if there's no tomorrow by eating unnutritious foods, getting inadequate rest, and not paying attention to matters of the heart is disastrous, too.

Creating a lifestyle that supports meaning in living and balances mental, emotional, spiritual, and physical needs is a better way to go.

Although the term "wellness" is overused and often misunderstood, the concept holds valuable and useful insights with regard to getting the most out of living.

Wellness is built on the foundation of developing a positive attitude toward overall health, personal responsibility, balance, and being true to oneself. Living flows naturally, gracefully, and meaningfully. Wellness is more than being healthy and free from illness and disease. John Travis, M.D., believes that "High-level wellness results from taking good care of your physical self, using your mind constructively, expressing your emotions effectively, channeling stress energies positively, being creatively involved with those around you, and being concerned about your physical and psychological environment."

SPICES for Life© is a comprehensive approach to wellness which features six different but interelated dimensions. SPICES stands for **S**ocial, **P**hysical, **I**ntellectual, **C**areer, **E**motional, and **S**piritual well-being. Each of these areas are equally important to living a well-rounded, good life, and equal attention should be given to developing and balancing them in life.

A person who is **socially** active and alive is one who is able to establish and maintain meaningful relationships with others. He or she is comfortable being and working with people from different age groups, cultures, and backgrounds. Socially aware people are knowledgeable of the issues affecting their community and work to improve their community by volunteering, voting, and being involved.

The **physical** dimension of wellness is much more than getting the right amount of exercise. It also means eating balanced, nutritious meals; maintaining proper body weight in relation to your frame size, and paying attention to safety (for example, wearing seat belts, preventing fires, locking doors, not drinking and driving). Physically well people don't get sick very often and make lifestyle choices that help prevent future health problems. This includes age-appropriate annual checkups, immunizations, and screening exams. In addition to concentration on the individual, choices and actions are taken to protect the earth's environment by recycling, reusing, renewing, and reducing the amount of resources used.

Intellectually healthy people tend to engage in creative, stimulating mental activities. They are active problem-solvers and learn from their mistakes. They set short- and long-term goals and take steps to achieve their goals. Intellectually alert people are open to new ideas and are open to change. Also included is the interest in current events, arts, and entertainment. Curiosity, an interest in learning, and the development of new skills throughout life are also signs of intellectually well people.

Career development is another part of being well-rounded. Having goals or directions in life are as important as taking the steps to achieve these goals. The satisfaction gained by one's work, whether in school, on the job, or at home, and the degree of enrichment that is felt, are measures of career health. A positive attitude toward one's work and maintaining balance is also important.

Emotional well-being is related to one's awareness and acceptance of feelings and the ability to express feelings in a positive, productive manner. Emotionally healthy people generally experience and appropriately express a wide range of emotions and feelings. They also accept others' expressions of feelings. They feel positive about themselves and are enthusiastic about their lives and selves and are able to cope with stress. Emotionally stable people are responsible (that is, are able to respond) to emotional issues.

Spiritually well people are involved in the ongoing development of a purpose and philosophy of life. They are involved in the internal development of a personal set of values, beliefs, and ethics. They strive to live by these and acknowledge and appreciate the depth and expanse of life. Their spiritual nature supports and enhances their mental and emotional self.

Yoga supports, enhances, and encourages wellness at all levels by bringing a sense of balance and harmony to daily living. This is especially true when care and attention is regularly devoted to each of the dimensions of wellness.

fifteen

Energy Answers

Why does it seem so hard to have just the right amount of energy? We are either wired and on the go all the time or feel tired and totally out of energy. It's no wonder that our lives sometimes feel empty and we lose sight of meaningful relationships, situations, and circumstances.

Life is lived on fast-forward as we try to cram more into an already packed day. More meetings to attend, more responsibilities to handle, more work to do in less time, more volunteering, and more exercises to fit in. We push ourselves to do more. Our employers, family, friends, civic, social, and religious organizations push us. In other words, there just isn't enough time and energy to go around. This leaves us feeling incredibly busy and makes it seem impossible to slow down and get some rest. In fact, wholesome, normal rest begins to feel foreign and can bring on guilty feelings.

At other times, we feel so fatigued that it's too hard to think, move, or do much of anything. We let ourselves get so tired that we can't even sleep.

If you recognize yourself in these situations, here are some "energy answers" to help you get back on track. Creating more personal energy will require you to make lifestyle changes. Doing so will cause an amazing ripple effect throughout your life which is well worth the time and trouble.

Coping with Change

Understanding and coming to terms with the change process is a great help in coping with planned change as well as in dealing with unwanted, unplanned change. Rather than feeling confused and abused by change, you'll be better equipped to handle it if you know what to expect. Cynthia Scott has identified the common stages of change to be denial, resistance, exploration, and commitment. Integrating Desktop Yoga into your day can be used to illustrate these concepts.

Denial

"Who needs it? Certainly not me!" "How could Desktop Yoga have all those benefits?" are sentiments often voiced by a person in denial. At the same time, the aches and pains of working are being ignored. Making the connection between leaving work with a headache and a stiff back day after day is not associated with sitting slumped over in the chair with poor posture. A sore neck is not believed to be related to holding the telephone receiver between your shoulder and ear throughout the day. Apathy often goes hand-in-hand with denial.

Resistance

Recognizing resistance is easy. "I don't have time for this nonsense." "I'll look stupid and people will make fun of me." "What if I can't do it or it makes me feel worse?" "For heaven's sake, the last thing I want to do is let my stomach relax and pooch out when breathing in." "Besides, I'm not flexible." "No way!"

As resistance takes its course, feelings of loss are often experienced. It's not uncommon to slip into anger, guilt, and blame as changes are taking place. After all, adapting to something new means that it is necessary to let go of something old and familiar. Feelings of grief are normal and necessary in this stage.

Exploration

Resistance finally gives way to exploration and is characterized by a period of experimentation. With acceptance comes an explosion of new ideas. These ideas, more often than not, are chaotic in nature. Here's how it works: Desktop Yoga is tried in a haphazard manner. Some days you do it in the mornings, other times it's done in the afternoon. Then there are periods of time when it isn't done at all. Perhaps the focus is solely on the postures designed for the back while excluding the ones for the face, neck, arms, and legs. "Maybe Desktop Yoga will end all my troubles." "I think I'll take a yoga class. Better yet, I'll quit this lousy job and move to India for a year or two." This stage is both exciting and very disorganized.

Commitment

Commitment is the final stage in the change process. During this period, the new thought, feeling, or behavior becomes integrated and begins to feel natural and normal. "I can't imagine not doing Desktop Yoga. It really helps my energy and I feel so much better."

Warning: no matter whether the change is perceived to be positive or negative, it is important and necessary go through each and every stage. This will insure a healthy, long-lasting change. It isn't necessary, however, to spend months and months in each of the stages. Passing through them is all it takes.

Fifty-three Energy Answers

1. Eat nutritious foods that are fresh and wholesome. Likewise, processed foods that are high in fat, sugar, or salt will deplete your energy—and make you fat. Try to listen to your body, so you'll know when you've eaten enough.

2. Practice relaxation exercises and meditation to restore your well-being significantly and substantially.

3. Build stress relief into every day instead of waiting until it's too late. Get a massage, take a warm bath, light a candle, spend time in nature, get physical, listen to enjoyable music, spend time with family, friends, and pets, laugh and have a good time.

4. Develop a positive mental attitude. Worrying is a mental and physical drain that robs energy. Take things one at a time, stay in the moment, and avoid obsessing about the future.

5. Stay on a regular schedule to take advantage of your natural daily and monthly rhythms. Establish regular times for eating, sleeping, and exercising. The routine will reward you with stability, balance, and endurance.

6. Take care of yourself so you don't get sick or injured. Prevent problems before they happen by eating nutritious foods, balancing adequate rest with exercise, getting a flu shot, having regular checkups, avoid drinking and driving, install smoke alarms, and wear your seat belt. Ignoring these things can result in time-consuming and stressful illnesses and accidents.

7. Breathe diaphragmatically. It can help you calm down, think more clearly, improve your memory, relieve the knotted feeling in your gut, and improve heart function, circulation, and digestion.

8. Start coping with change. It's all around us so stop fighting it. Learn to gracefully negotiate the natural reactions that result from change. They are denial, resistance, exploration, and commitment.

9. Do one thing at a time. Focus on the moment. Don't get caught up in the past or future.

10. Do it right, not over.

11. Grow. Take advantage of training.

12. Laugh.

13. Take a walk.

14. Be around positive people. Avoid whiners.

15. If you really don't like your work or work environment, find something new.

16. Avoid too much caffeine, soda, alcohol, and junk food. Better yet, stop using the above. Don't smoke.

17. Get involved in your company's wellness program.

18. Try your company's Employee Assistance Program (EAP). They usually help with personal, financial, legal, and substance abuse problems.

19. Enjoy nature.

20. Move around. Take a ten-minute walk. Use the stairs instead of the elevator or escalator.

21. Smile.

22. Get some fresh air.

23. Manage your time wisely.

24. Plan ahead. Be prepared.

25. Balance work with an active home and play life.

26. Get enough rest. Take a nap.

27. Say a prayer.

28. Don't get caught up in gossip or negative thinking.

29. It's all a game. Be a team player and play well with others.

30. If you're in a hole, quit digging deeper.

31. Go for results, not activity.

32. Schedule time for yourself.

33. Don't be your own worst enemy.

34. Take a relaxation break and practice the activities described in chapter 10 regarding power naps.

35. Remember that whatever is happening is only temporary. That goes for both the little picture and the big picture.

36. Keep your perspective.

37. If you are going to laugh about it in ten years, why not laugh now?

38. Focus. Leave work at work and home life at home.

39. Don't skip meals.

40. Have fun.

41. Say yes when you can, and no when you can't.

42. Drink plenty of water.

43. Enjoy the journey and let the destination take care of itself.

44. Pick your battles carefully.

45. Get over it.

46. Want what you have.

47. Simplify your life.

48. Get to know yourself. Be yourself.

49. Love yourself. Love others.

50. Hum, sing, dance.

51. Wear comfortable shoes.

52. Exercise regularly.

53. Do Desktop Yoga.

In short, your stamina and vitality will grow in strength when you learn to cope with change and take meaningful time for yourself.

sixteen

Stress Survival Skills

*G*oing through life's adjustments and changes can add unwanted stress, causing unhappiness, sickness, poor relationships, and lack of energy. Stress can be felt whenever anything changes—positive or negative—and since it is impossible to escape, it becomes important to learn how to handle stress without distress.

Admit it, stress motivates us and even makes life juicy when handled appropriately. Would you really try your hardest on that report if you weren't afraid of the consequences of turning in an inferior one? Would you want to give up the feelings of joy and satisfaction that come from personal or professional accomplishments just to avoid the time, effort, and stress involved?

Ever since the early days of lions, tigers, and bears, the body has reacted to stress by preparing either to fight or flee. The heart automatically speeds up; stress hormones are released (adrenaline, norepinephrine, cortisol); pupils dilate; skin becomes pale; blood pressure rises; digestion, salivation, kidney, and liver functions slow; breathing becomes shallow and unrhythmic; and metabolic changes occur. These reactions take place when stress is experi-

117

enced, whether it is real or imagined. For instance, feeling afraid of getting chewed out by your boss will trigger the stress response and can be just as hard on you as the real thing.

When appropriate, this reaction is a lifesaver, especially when you are being followed in a dark alley and need to get away or fight for your life. Yet it turns into trouble if this is the constant state of affairs in your body. Stress damages the heart, creates chronic muscle tension, disrupts digestion and elimination, and can lead to mental and emotional problems.

Let's Get Personal: Identifying Your Physical, Psychological, and Environmental Sources of Stress

The causes of stress are either controllable or uncontrollable. The trick is to learn how to control the controllable and figure out how to cope with the uncontrollable. The first step is to learn to identify the sources of your stress by determining whether the source is environmental, psychological, or physical. Stress is an individual matter for everyone. What sends one person over the edge is regarded as a challenge for someone else. How you react to stress is very personal. No matter what triggers stress for you, the important thing is to recognize it and break the cycle.

Take advantage of the following checklists to discover more about yourself.

Many of the major symptoms of stress are physical. To name a few, there are headaches, tight shoulders, a knot in the stomach, and insomnia. Problems such as these are distracting, uncomfortable, and time-consuming. Begin by checking off your common physical reactions and results of stress.

Physical Symptoms

_____ Headaches
_____ Sweaty palms
_____ Sleep problems (too much or too little)
_____ Fatigue
_____ Back pain

_____ Stomachaches/indigestion

_____ Skin rashes

_____ Dry mouth

_____ Muscle tension

_____ Diarrhea or constipation

_____ Cold hands or feet

_____ Grinding teeth

_____ Eating too much or too little

_____ Drug abuse (alcohol, tobacco, prescription, and/or illegal drugs)

Add your own _____

_____

Take Charge

Read the example below, and then use the following worksheet to help you think through possible solutions to smooth out your stress.

Physical stressor:
"Not being able to sleep at night."

Possible causes:
"I drink coffee and soda all day."

Is it controllable?　　　__X__ Yes　　　_____ No

Personal reaction:
"I feel upset when I can't sleep and then I can't concentrate very well the next day."

Is my reaction controllable?　　__X__ Yes　　　_____ No

Possible solution. What resources will help? When can I start?
"I could stop drinking caffeine after 5 P.M. I could also listen to a relaxation tape to help me get to sleep."

Benefits and rewards:
"My sleep will be more restful and I'll have more usable energy."

1. Physical stressor _____

_____

Possible causes _____

_____

Is it controllable?   _____ Yes   _____ No

Personal reaction _____

_____

Is my reaction controllable?   _____ Yes   _____ No

Possible solution. What resources will help? When can I start?

_____

_____

Benefits and rewards _____

_____

2. Physical stressor _____

_____

Possible causes _____

_____

Is it controllable?   _____ Yes   _____ No

Personal reaction _____

_____

Is my reaction controllable?   _____ Yes   _____ No

Possible solution. What resources will help? When can I start?

_____

_____

Benefits and rewards _____

_____

Stress is also derived from **psychological sources** and can be internally based. Anger, impatience, depression, and boredom are examples. Check off a few of your "favorite" emotional and mental symptoms.

Emotional Symptoms

_____ Feeling edgy
_____ Depression
_____ Nervousness
_____ Crying
_____ Feeling pressure
_____ Anger
_____ Apathy
_____ Dissatisfaction
_____ Tension
_____ Fear
_____ Embarrassment
_____ Guilt
_____ Losing your temper
_____ Withdrawing from others
_____ Being argumentative, critical, or bossy

Add your own _____

_____

Mental Symptoms

_____ Confusion
_____ Forgetfulness or memory loss
_____ Constant worry
_____ Boredom
_____ Indecision
_____ Irrational thoughts
_____ Making mistakes, errors
_____ Unwanted thoughts
_____ Decrease in attention span
_____ Feeling scattered
_____ Obsessing
_____ Being easily distracted

Add your own _____

_____

Take Charge

Read the example below describing a psychological stressor, and then use the worksheet to generate ideas that will be helpful to you.

Psychological stressor:
"I've been worried and irritated and now I feel guilty for snapping at my friend."

Possible causes:
"I'm worried about all the downsizing that is going on. I took my frustrations out on my friend."

Is it controllable?   _X_ Yes   _____ No

Personal reaction:
"I feel overwhelmed by my worries and guilty for snapping at my friend."

Is my reaction controllable?   __X__ Yes   _____ No

Possible solution. What resources will help? When can I start?
"I could apologize to my friend and ask her for some advice to solve my worries. We could go for a walk and burn off some steam."

Benefits and rewards:
"I'll feel better about myself and my friendship will be strengthened."

1. Psychological stressor _____
_____

Possible causes _____
_____

Is it controllable?   _____ Yes   _____ No

Personal reaction _____
_____

Is my reaction controllable?   _____ Yes   _____ No

Possible solution. What resources will help? When can I start?
_____
_____

Benefits and rewards _____
_____

2. Psychological stressor _____
_____

Possible causes _____
_____

Is it controllable? _____ Yes _____ No

Personal reaction _____

_____

Is my reaction controllable? _____ Yes _____ No

Possible solution. What resources will help? When can I start?

_____

_____

Benefits and rewards _____

_____

Environmental Stress

This comes from reactions to outside sources in the shape of people, places, circumstances, and events. A few examples are traffic jams, loud and distracting noises, people who get on your nerves, and deadlines. Review the following situations and mark the ones that bother you.

Situational Reactions and Symptoms

_____ Deadlines
_____ Traffic jams or parking problems
_____ Too much to do in too little time
_____ Having to wait in lines or for someone
_____ People who irritate you
_____ Being late
_____ Financial problems
_____ Auto and home equipment breakdowns
_____ Loud and distracting noises
_____ Losing things (keys, money, etc.)
_____ Weather-related problems (ice, rain, heat, etc.)

_____ Taxes
_____ Unsatisfying work
_____ Problems of family and friends

Add your own _____

Take Charge

List a few of your environmental stresses here, decide whether they are controllable or not, and design a solution.

Environmental stressor:
"I hate my job and it gets on my nerves. My back kills me by the end of the day."

Possible causes:
"I hardly ever know what I'm doing; there is too much to remember."
"Poor posture, lack of stretch breaks, improper ergonomics."

Is it controllable?   _____ Yes   _X_ No *"I have to work."*

Personal reaction:
"I feel frustrated and overwhelmed."
"I feel achy, tired, and stressed out."

Is my reaction controllable?   _X_ Yes   _____ No

Possible solution. What resources will help? When can I start?
"I'll ask my supervisor for additional training and take notes to help me remember."
"Tomorrow, I'll do some Desktop Yoga to keep my shoulders and back from aching. Breathing deeply will probably settle my nerves and I'll finally get around to adjusting the height of my chair to improve my posture."

Benefits and rewards:
"My energy will improve and I'll feel much better."

1. Environmental stressor _____
_____

Possible causes _____
_____

Is it controllable? _____ Yes _____ No

Personal reaction _____
_____

Is my reaction controllable? _____ Yes _____ No

Possible solution. What resources will help? When can I start?
_____
_____

Benefits and rewards _____
_____

2. Environmental stressor _____
_____

Possible causes _____
_____

Is it controllable? _____ Yes _____ No

Personal reaction _____
_____

Is it controllable? _____ Yes _____ No

Possible solution. What resources will help? When can I start?

_____

_____

Benefits and rewards _____

_____

Handling Stress

The importance of handling stress cannot be emphasized enough. Fortunately, stress can be reduced and unhealthy reactions can be controlled to a certain degree. **DARE** to improve your ability to handle stress by practicing the following effective coping techniques.

DARE to Relax© includes: **D** = Diet; **A** = Attitude and Awareness, **R** = Rest and Relaxation; **E** = Exercise.[1]

Diet

Don't deprive yourself of essential nutrients, vitamins, and minerals that can help you reduce the effects of daily stress. Stress depletes your supply of vitamins A, B, and C, which can lead to having you feel irritable and tired. Calcium is essential for your central nervous system to function normally; without enough of it, your nerves become too easily excitable. If you consistently eat well-balanced meals, you can fortify and nourish yourself to guard against the harmful effects of stress. Here are some tips:

—Eat a nutritious breakfast.

—Choose fresh fruits, vegetables, and whole grains.

—Choose baked, boiled, or broiled food instead of fried.

_____

1. DARE to Relax © by Julie T. Lusk, M.Ed., LPC

—Cut down on excessive fat, salt, sugar, caffeine, additives, and preservatives.

—Get adequate fiber, protein, and carbohydrates.

—Maintain a healthy weight.

—Drink alcohol in moderation, if at all.

Attitude and Awareness

Research shows that between 60 and 80 percent of illnesses are the result of experiencing too much stress. Not being able to handle stress properly can decrease the effectiveness of your immune system. Become more aware of how you respond to tension and stress in your life and begin to make some adjustments. Are you responding appropriately? Could you be overreacting? Is it possible to avoid or change a situation that causes you anxiety? You may be able to avoid some of your headaches, stomachaches, and other problems by improving your awareness and making improvements in the ways you react to stress. Try laughing. Laughter is like internal jogging. It aids digestion, improves alertness and productivity by sending blood and oxygen to your brain, and increases the production of the body's catecholamines.

—Learn to accept situations you can't change; give in once in a while.

—Learn to communicate with others; talk your worries out.

—Take one thing at a time; don't take on too many changes at once.

—Manage your time more effectively; don't procrastinate.

—Be positive and realistic.

—Express your feelings in healthy ways.

—Create variety in your work.

—Do old things in new ways.

Rest and Relaxation

It is much easier to handle stress if you are rested and know how to remain calm. Getting seven to eight hours of sleep every night is essential. Although recreation and being diverted from stress (playing tennis, watching a movie, reading) is helpful, true relaxation is different. It involves giving yourself an honest break from activity and excess stimulation. Breathing deeply, smoothly, slowly, and from the diaphragm is relaxing. It sends a fresh supply of blood to the brain and throughout the body, oxygenates your system, and stimulates the vagus nerve, which slows down the heartbeat.

—Plan leisure time; take breaks.

—Spend time on a hobby; seek new interests.

—Schedule some quiet time alone every day; meditate; pray.

—Have fun, play, and laugh.

—Cut down on noise levels at home and work; turn the radio or television off.

Exercise

When under stress, there is an increase of adrenaline in the system as part of the flight or fight response. This can drain you of energy if not effectively released. Work off your stress positively with regular exercise. This can improve your productivity and increase your energy. Be sure to choose exercises that you enjoy.

Daily stress and strain commonly occurs and cannot be stopped or ignored. Taking time to identify your stressors, noticing your physical, mental, and emotional reactions to it, and finding healthy ways to handle stress, is well worth the time and effort. Doing so will lead to a more fulfilling and healthy life.

Twelve Yoga Secrets for Managing Stress

Every day, people come to yoga to learn how to lower stress and alleviate the damage caused by tension and strain. Fortunately, the act of practicing yoga fosters physical, mental, and emotional relaxation during the time that the postures and breathing techniques are performed. Better yet, the underlying philosophy and relaxed attitude continues beyond the time spent doing yoga, and begins to permeate other aspects of living.

1. Yoga increases your personal awareness. Increased awareness will enable you to recognize and notice tension as it occurs, and give you practical and useful actions and attitudes to reduce stress and replace it with relaxation. For example, you will be able to catch muscular tension and know how to relieve it before it creates muscular tightness and pain.

2. Yoga focuses on the body, mind, heart, and spirit. You've probably noticed how some people live almost exclusively in only one aspect of their being. Rather than living in balance and alignment, their perspective is limited. For instance, there are people who are entrenched in the intellectual realm, and ignore their bodies and their emotions. Others operate from their emotional center and don't take advantage of their minds and body. Then there are those who repress their emotions and concentrate their efforts on their bodies. Do you know people who spend all their time exercising and obsessing over food, so that they don't seem to have any other interests or relationships?

Yoga moves the body, awakens the mind, and opens the heart and spirit. You can do this by being aware of each movement, remembering to breathe, thinking of the benefits derived from the position, and noticing mental and emotional reactions resulting from the poses.

3. Yoga literally teaches the experience of total relaxation. It gives you the time and permission to let go and release physical tensions from the body. One way this is done is consciously to tense and release individual muscle groups. This demonstrates what tension actually feels like as well as what the experience of feeling relaxed is. When the body relaxes, the mind and emotions calm down, too. When you are able to recognize muscular tension while

driving, for example, you can remember to take a deep breath and do some shoulder rolls to relieve the tightness rather than let it turn into a headache.

4. Yoga teaches you how to use the correct amount of energy and effort to get the job done. It is unnecessary and counterproductive to overstretch your muscles and force yourself beyond your current capacity. This will help you stop being "your own worst enemy" by pushing yourself too hard.

5. Yoga activates the mind–body connection by bringing it to your conscious awareness. This can be done by mindfully coordinating the body movements with the breath. Doing so will have a positive effect on your health and well-being.

6. Full and complete breathing brings oxygen to the brain, which results in the ability to think more clearly, concentrate more closely, and assist with solving problems.

7. Yoga helps prevent health problems by massaging, cleansing, and oxygenating each and every cell, organ, and gland in the body. Illness and accidents can be prevented and the immune system is strengthened. Stressful living leads to sickness and getting sick is stressful, wastes time, and generates unnecessary expenses and hassles. Staying healthy in the first place by managing stress is invaluable.

8. Living in the moment is taught in yoga. You are encouraged to return your attention to the present each time the mind wanders from the movement or breath. Wasting time by reliving the past or worrying about the future is discouraged. Getting the most out of life by living in the moment is positive and creates the potential for a wonderful future.

9. Self-acceptance is mastered and self-esteem naturally increases through the practice of yoga when the proper attitude toward achievement is maintained. It is not helpful to be either critical or complimentary toward your ability to do yoga. It is much more important to accept yourself for who and how you are. Being yourself is enough. It is a lot less stressful if you are able to stop putting yourself down all the time and if you can stop punishing yourself for not measuring up. It really doesn't matter how flexible you are. It is much more important to be aware of your capabilities and accept yourself.

10. Yoga emphasizes ethical behavior through the five *yamas,* or disciplines, as taught by Patanjali. They give us guidelines to follow in the relationships and attitudes toward people and things outside ourselves.

The first one is nonviolence in actions, thoughts, and words. In other words, not harming anything. Kindness, thoughtfulness, and being considerate of oneself, other people, and things are highly valued. This approach softens relationships and fosters love.

Truthfulness is the second yama. Life is a lot simpler and less confusing when you are being honest with yourself and others. Honesty, however, should never bring harm to others. Brutal truth can hurt and should be avoided. Being true to yourself and following the other yamas will help you be true to others.

Not stealing is the third yama. This includes not taking the possessions, ideas, or anything else from others. Refrain from taking advantage of people or situations.

Moral conduct and moving toward truth by acting responsibly is the fourth discipline. Abstinence is associated with this yama, and further suggests that we form relationships that are built on the highest truths.

The last yama is to not be greedy and to use only that which is necessary. Exploitation is discouraged.

11. Developing your spirituality is an important yoga principle. Take the time to identify and develop your beliefs and values and live by them. Yoga is not a religion, although this is a common misperception. It does encourage you to develop a strong relationship with the divine in whatever manner you choose. There are many forms and paths that can be followed to accomplish this. Some people get the most out of formal religious organizations while others prefer the informal approach. Prayer, meditation, and enjoying nature are a few favorites.

12. Yoga will help you develop a relationship to life and living that is positive, productive, and enhances health. It will help you loosen your attachment to results and expectations and open you up to thoughts and feelings of freedom and possibilities. The sense of acceptance, contentment, and fulfillment will begin to replace feelings of dissatisfaction toward yourself and others.

Resources

This book has featured yoga-based postures that can be done sitting at a computer station or desk. There are, however, thousands more yoga postures that are designed to be done standing, sitting, or lying on the floor. The best way to learn yoga is to join a class, and there are many styles of yoga to choose from. Check with your local colleges, churches, hospitals, the Y, athletic clubs, and recreation centers.

You will find yoga classes that emphasize slow, gentle movements, while others are vigorous and strenuous. Some teachers stress precision and alignment; others don't. There are those that tend to be physical in nature while others have a more spiritual flavor. Look for a class that suits your temperament and needs.

Before choosing, spend a little time talking to various teachers (if you are fortunate to have a choice) and ask them what their classes are like. Be sure to ask about their training, how long they have been doing yoga, and how long they have been teaching. Although it is not a guarantee, you may be better off finding a teacher who is certified. Unfortunately, all the teacher certification courses have different standards, and some are better than others. It is possible to find good teachers who are not certified and there are lots of certified teachers with limited experience.

In general, books on yoga do not go out of date. After all, yoga itself dates back thousands of years. Here are some resources to investigate. I've starred my favorites.

Books

Birch, Beryl Bender. *Power Yoga.* New York: Simon and Schuster, 1995.

Carrico, Mara. *Yoga Journal's Yoga Basics.* New York: Henry Holt and Company, Inc., 1997.

Christensen, Alice and the American Yoga Association. *20 Minute Yoga Workouts.* New York: Ballantine Books, 1995.

Couch, Jean. *The Runner's Yoga Book.* California: Rodmell Press, 1990.

Desikachar, T.K.V. *The Heart of Yoga.* California: Rodmell Press, 1990.

Devi, Indra. *Renew Your Life Through Yoga.* New York: Warner Books, 1963.

———. *Yoga for Americans.* Englewood Cliffs, NJ: Prentice Hall, 1959.

Farhi, Donna. *The Breathing Book: Good Health and Vitality Through Essential Breath Work.* New York: Henry Holt and Company, 1996.

Folan, Lilias. *Lilias, Yoga & Your Life.* New York: Collier Books, 1981.

Gach, Michael Reed. *Acu-Yoga.* Japan: Japan Publications, 1991.

Hewitt, James. *The Complete Yoga Book.* New York: Schocken Books, 1978.

Hittleman, Richard. *Guide to Yoga Meditation.* New York: Bantam, 1969.

———. *Yoga 28 Day Exercise Plan.* New York: Workman Publishing Co., 1969.

Iyengar, B.K.S. *Light on Yoga.* New York: Schocken Books, 1979.

Janakananda Saraswati, Swami. *Yoga, Tantra & Meditation.* New York: Ballantine Books, 1975.

Kent, Howard. *Yoga Made Easy.* Pennsylvania: Quarto Publishing, 1993.

Lasater, Judith. *Relax and Renew.* California: Rodmell Press, 1995.

Leggett, T. *Yoga and Zen: Meetings of Cloth and Stone.* Boston: Routledge and Kegan Paul, 1982.

Lusk, Julie T. *30 Scripts for Relaxation, Imagery and Inner Healing, Vols. 1 and 2.* Duluth, MN: Whole Person Press, 1992, 1993.

Rama, Swami. *Lectures on Yoga.* Honesdale, PA: Himalayan International Institute of Yoga Science and Philosophy, 1979.

Samskrti, and J. Franks. *Hatha Yoga.* Honesdale, PA: International Institute of Yoga Science and Philosophy, 1978.

Satchidananda, Swami. *Integral Yoga Hatha.* New York: Holt, Rinehart, and Winston, 1970.

Scaravelli, Vanda. *Awakening the Spine.* New York: HarperCollins, 1991.

Schatz, Mary Pullig. *Back Care Basics.* California: Rodmell Press, 1992.

Schiffmann, Erich. *Yoga: The Spirit and Practice of Moving Into Stillness.* New York: Pocket Books, 1996.

Stearn, Jesse. *Yoga, Youth and Reincarnation.* New York: Bantam, 1965.

Strutt, Malcolm. *Wholistic Health & Living Yoga.* Boulder Creek: The University of the Trees Press, 1977.

Thompson, Judi. *Healthy Pregnancy the Yoga Way.* Garden City, NY: Dolphin Books, 1977.

Tobias, Maxine and Mary Stewart. *Stretch and Relax.* Tucson, AZ: The Body Press, 1985.

Van Lysebeth, Andre. *Yoga Self-Taught.* New York: Barnes and Noble, 1971.

Vishnudevananda, Swami. *The Complete Illustrated Book of Yoga.* New York: Bell Publishing, 1960.

Weinrib, David and Jo Ann Weinrib. *A Book of Yoga: The Body Temple.* New York: Quadrangle/The New York Times Book Co., 1974.

Ward, Susan Winter. *Yoga for the Young at Heart.* Santa Barbara, CA: Capra Press, 1994.

Videos

Yoga Journal produces excellent yoga videos. They have videos for beginners, relaxation, strength, flexibility, energy, and meditation. Call 1-800-436-YOGA (9642).

Beginning:

Ward, Susan Winter. *Yoga for the Young at Heart,* 1994. 1-800-558-YOGA (9642).

Intermediate:

Rich, Tracey, and Ganga White. *Total Yoga.* White Lotus Yoga Foundation, 1994. 1-800-544-FLOW (3569).

Advanced:

Rich, Tracey, and Ganga White. *Vinyasa Yoga, The Flow Series.* White Lotus Yoga Foundation, 1990. 1-800-544-FLOW (3569).

Periodicals

Yoga International. Call 1-800-253-6243 to subscribe.

Yoga Journal. Call 1-800-436-9642 to subscribe.

Index

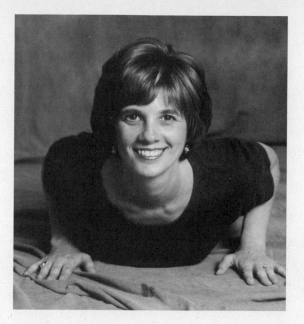

*J*ulie T. Lusk, M.Ed., designs and implements nationally recognized mind/body and wellness programs for businesses, medical centers, communities, and individuals. She enjoys sharing realistic methods to cope with stress, improve performance, and feel better emotionally, physically, and mentally.

As a certified yoga teacher, Julie has taught yoga since 1977. She earned her yoga teacher certification through the White Lotus Foundation and has broadened her training by undertaking numerous advanced courses.

In an effort to relieve stressful working conditions for computer users and other workers, Julie has modified over 100 yoga postures so they can easily be done while working or at a computer station. These useful exercises, as well as stress management and wellness strategies, are presented in her book, *Desktop Yoga*™.

Julie is the editor and author of the popular books *30 Scripts for Relaxation, Imagery and Inner Healing, Volumes One and Two*. Her cassette, *Refreshing Journeys*, is a guided imagery sampler which is done in her warm and gentle style. These books and tapes are available through Whole Person Press, Duluth, MN.

Professionally, she has worked in health care management, higher education, and community organizing and has helped thousands of people through her volunteer work. She is currently the Regional Director of the Mercy Holistic Center.

Julie is available as a keynote speaker, to customize seminars, as a consultant to corporate, collegiate, and community groups, and for individual appointments. Client list, references, and fees are available upon request. JTLusk@aol.com.